MW00784420

# Iron Ball, Wooden Staff, Empty Hands

# Iron Ball, Wooden Staff, Empty Hands

## Understanding Structure, Flow, and Maneuver in Martial Arts

### Caylor Adkins

*Pine Winds Press*

An imprint of Idyll Arbor, Inc.
39129 264th Ave SE, Enumclaw, WA 98022
www.PineWindsPress.com

Pine Winds Press Editor: Thomas M. Blaschko

Photographs: Kerry Copeland and Thomas M. Blaschko
Art Work: Michael Duray, Dave Shaver, and Brian Borrello

© 2011 Idyll Arbor, Inc.

International copyright protection is reserved under Universal Copyright Convention and bilateral copyright relations of the USA. All rights reserved, which includes the right to reproduce this book or any portions thereof in any form whatsoever except as provided by the relevant copyright laws.

ISBN 9780937663134

**Library of Congress Cataloging-in-Publication Data**

Adkins, Caylor.
  Iron ball, wooden staff, empty hands : understanding structure, flow, and maneuver in martial arts / Caylor Adkins.
      p. cm.
  Includes bibliographical references and index.
  ISBN 978-0-937663-13-4 (alk. paper)
  1. Martial arts--Training.  I. Title.
  GV1102.7.T7A45 2010
  796.815--dc22

                                                2010033673

# Dedication

*To Carol, who has my back, who covers my six*
*To my instructors over the years, and most of all to Mr. Tsutomu Ohshima*
*To my training partners over the years*
*To my students over the years*
*Who have all taught me so very much*

THANK YOU

# Acknowledgements

In 1966 I experienced a severely broken neck with a subsequent steady physical degradation.

So a heartfelt thank you to Steve Bankes, Rolfer, and to Karen Parry, magic chiropractor, whose battlefield repairs over the years kept me going.

A special thanks to Doctor Jeffery Wang whose surgical skill in 2000 gave me back the martial arts life I had feared lost to me.

To Tom Blaschko, an editor with near-mythic patience and an insightful martial artist who brings that understanding to dealing with my chaotic style of writing; a thousand thanks, Tom.

# Contents

# Preface

This started as a personal book, organizing thoughts and observations from my initial foray into the martial arts in 1957 to the present.

Five years ago, as I started to teach what I had written, it became a collaboration of sorts as I explain below.

The text of this book started with lists of things to remember and things to try working on once my neck problems were resolved. This was in the time period leading up to my surgery (1998-2000) and during the rehabilitation period (2000-2002).

After the rehab I started working out in earnest and upon resuming serious ball work found that it greatly enhanced my supposedly adequate physical recovery.

Applying new understanding from the ball work to many of the list items was very productive. I started to outline my new insights, intensively work on them, and communicate them to my training partners. This book is the result.

Along the way my emphasis and conclusions continually changed, but the effort of putting thoughts down on a computer clarified my thinking a lot and was very helpful in guiding my practice.

Considering the potential of the ball practice, this book is far from complete, but this is about as far as I can go with my current understanding and I believe this is a reasonable introduction to using a ball as part of martial arts practice.

I am rapidly not getting any younger, so I need to stop focusing on the ball and start working the rest of my list items.

I would welcome any insights, positive, negative, or mixed from any who also work with the ball.

There are several ways to represent the sounds of Oriental languages with Western letters. I have tried to use the words that will be most familiar to you, but where I have quoted material from another source, I kept the representation that was in the original text. It is probably enough to know the following equivalences to understand this text.

Chi can also be represented as Qi (as in Qi Gong), Ki (the usual Japanese pronunciation), and Ji (often used in Tai Ji).

Tai Chi Chuan can also be written as Tai Ji Quan.

Kung Fu is sometimes Gungfu and Chi Gong is the same as Qi Gong.

# 1. Introduction

I wrote this book to show how practicing with an iron ball complemented by weapons can enhance the practice of almost any martial artist.

Martial arts practice, for the most part, is divided between external styles and internal styles. Some of you reading this will practice biomechanical external styles, others the energetic internal styles, and some the styles that are a blend of the two approaches. I'm sure you will find some things in here where you say, "I know that. It's so obvious." Other places you'll be saying, "That sounds like total BS." I hope there will also be some places where you say, "interesting" or "damn, that's a good idea."

Considering the wide spectrum of martial arts practice, there are large numbers of important goals and objectives for the participants; probably many more than one could pursue in a lifetime. There are, however, many significant, important goals and objectives for which the ball practice is particularly well suited. That's why I am using the term "Big Deal."

A Big Deal is one of the significant principles and concepts in the martial arts. It may not be a Big Deal for everybody, but I hope that through this book you'll come to agree that anybody's Big Deal is worth studying, even if it's only to understand how to defeat them.

Some Big Deals receive way more "press" than others, deservedly so in most cases. I hope you will decide to pay extra attention to the concepts I indicate are Big Deals. There is usually a good payoff.

## Internal vs. External

I personally am basically an external martial arts practitioner but actually I find very little conflict between the internal and external rationales when describing what occurs in executing technique. It does take some study to "translate" internal energetic style terminology into biomechanical external style terminology, but it is time well spent. Many times I have been led to some very rewarding insights by the more intuitive direction of an internal practitioner who "connected the dots." Sometimes pointing out dots I was unaware of. See the appendices for some internal terminology samples.

Whether you choose an external or internal path really comes down to your motives for training in the first place. If you want something elegant, intellectually challenging, and eventually combat effective, the internal styles have great appeal. If you like a very physical training with a pretty quick combat ability, the external styles are a good bet.

Combat-wise there are some exceptions to this generalization. Within some of the internal styles there are a few intensely combat-oriented factions that produce quick results, and some of the external styles have a slow, step-by-step-by-step instructional process that is anything but quick to develop practical combat ability.

Asian martial arts have internal, external, and blended styles containing the entire broad range of energetic and biomechanical training.

Traditional Western martial arts such as boxing, wrestling, fencing, quarter-staff, etc. certainly fall into the external model. Boxing, for example, emphasizes punching with the whole body and not just the arm. From the feet to top of the head and ends of their fists a boxer's whole body is engaged and this is based on a thorough grounding in biomechanics.

Internal or external, whatever your initial choice was, motives can change. External style to internal style or vice versa are well-traveled paths. Perhaps the blended styles came from an acknowledgement of the desirability or even the necessity of studying both. One thing is certain: no one has the whole truth.

## Benefits of the Iron Ball

There are many objectives for people training in the martial arts: combat ability, basic self-defense, sport competition, health, recreation, character enhancement, vocational requirements or opportunities, etc.

My own bias is primarily for combat ability. The other benefits do come, but as a bonus. I feel that emphasizing real combat as the end game is the ultimate incentive for reaching the deepest understanding possible for you.

I did not want to write something that was academic, overly technical, or formal. This is not meant to be comprehensive or profound, just a narrowly focused presentation of material that has really benefited me and my fellow practitioners and that I would like to share.

Obviously, those with different backgrounds will have different problems and questions and thus different insights. Whatever the background, I feel that training with the ball and weapons will pay valuable dividends and enhance the understanding of martial arts practitioners.

In this book I show the value of the ball practice for both biomechanical and energetic approaches. Whichever is your primary emphasis, you can use the ball practice to work on your emphasis and gain insight into the complementary principles.

Training with the ball benefits both internal and external models. Both models require good structure and whole-body coordination, or form, or proper physical mechanics, or whatever it may be called to effectively execute technique.

Training with the ball is an effective tool for enhancing and integrating good structure with whole-body coordination.

## My Background

I have practiced martial arts since 1957: Shotokan karate the entire time, western boxing about 20 years and much more briefly Judo, Tai Chi Chuan, and Jeet Kune Do. Also, like most long-time practitioners, I have researched, observed, and "sampled" various other styles and arts.

## Background for Iron Ball Practice

I began the rudiments of this practice in 1964. My brother, Curt, spent several years in Taiwan during the 1960s studying the Chinese language. He also practiced some martial arts, primarily Long Fist Wushu with Han Ch'ing T'ang. Pursuing this interest he obtained a number of martial arts books. Among these were two that I particularly liked, both originally published in the 1920s. One by

Lu Wen Wei was entitled *Illustrated Explanation of Ball Exercises for Health* (*Nung Wan Jian Shen Tu Shuo*). This book depicts an internal style, quite complex and considerably outside my background, but absolutely intriguing. Check the appendices for a sample of this book's complexity. The other book, a set of two actually, was by Wan Lai Sheng entitled *Compendium of Internal and External Martial Arts* (*Wushu Nei Wai Gong Zonghui*). Volume one was subtitled "External Skills"; volume two was "Internal Skills." Volume one contained the staff form presented in this book. Volume two had some ball commentary (see appendices).

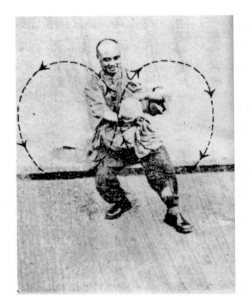

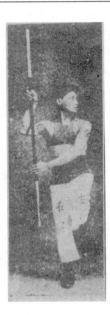

**Figure 1: Lu Wen Wei demonstrating Ball Posture One from *Illustrated Explanation of Ball Exercises for Health.***

**Figure 2: Wan Lai Sheng demonstrating techniques with a staff from *Compendium of Internal and External Martial Arts.***

Lu Wen Wei, trained in Wu Chi boxing and Tai Chi boxing. His multiple centers concept is (for me at least) the most unusual, challenging, and potentially rewarding idea in this book.

Quoting from his book:

My father was very disciplined regarding physical culture and never tired of constant training. He had a number of wooden and metal balls arrayed on a rack, the large ones about a foot in diameter, the middle ones five or six inches, and the small ones three to four inches. I also trained with them for three to four years, morning and night, and never tired of them. As a young man my father trained Xing Yi boxing and from this training derived two techniques, which he applied to ball training, zan and fan.

Some years ago I commenced training in Wu Ji boxing and Tai Ji boxing and, as my training progressed, I began to use the ball to replace the hand techniques. I devised twelve patterns that initiate with zan and then become fan and another 24 patterns that initiate with fan and change to zan. In this book the first twelve patterns are zan; the final 24 patterns are fan.

Fan and zan are discussed in detail on page 115 of this book. Web sites about Wu Ji and Tai Ji boxing are included in the appendices.

Wan Lai Sheng's experience is described in the biography taken from the Ziranmen Kung Fu Academy.[1]

Wan Lai Sheng is one of the legendary figures of Chinese Wushu. Born in Wuchang city, Hubei, Wan began his study of the martial arts at the age of seventeen, learning Shaolin Liu He boxing from Master Zhou Xin Zou. Looking to increase his skill and knowledge, Wan studied with just about every master he could find in the Beijing area. After graduating from Beijing Agricultural University, he tracked down Du Xin Wu, holder of the Zi Ran Men lineage and was accepted as his disciple.

---

[1] Article used with the permission of the Ziranmen Kung Fu Academy, http://www.ziranmen.com/wanlaisheng/wanlaisheng.php

Wan finally mastered the theories and practice of the Zi Ran Men school after seven years of concentrated study. Still hungry for knowledge, Wan absorbed the teachings of Xing Yi, Ba Gua, Luohan boxing, Wudang Tai Chi, Monkey style and Shaolin Luo Han Fist from Liu Ba Chuan, Wang Xiang Zhi, Wang Rong Biao, Ancestor Liu, and many others.

At this time Wan was asked to write a series of articles for the Beijing *Morning News*. Eventually the series was published as a book titled *A Collection of Reviews on Wushu*. It was the first book of its kind — drawing together and explaining all the different styles of Wushu.

In the same year, 1928, the first National Wushu Contest was held in Nanjing. Although the tournament was eventually halted due to the excessive injuries suffered by the fighters, Wan Lai Sheng was recognized as the preeminent martial artist in attendance.

Previously, Zi Ran Men had only been passed down to one disciple per generation. Under Du Din Wu's instructions, however, Wan begin to openly teach this style of boxing. Due to his skill and commitment, Zi Ran Men became famous, with schools rapidly developing nationwide.

Together with his cousin Wan Lai Ping and his friends Gu Ru Zhang, Li Xian Wu, and Fu Zhen Song [he] traveled to Guangzhou where he became director of the Guangzhou-Guangxi Wushu Academy. This has become a legendary event in the history of Chinese Wushu, known as Five Tigers Going South.

Wan Lai Sheng came to earn the title of "Big Dipper" — meaning that his skill level reached all the way up to the heavens. This is a very special accolade, as there can be only one "Big Dipper." This title wasn't just earned for his fighting skill; it also recognized Wan's study and understanding of literature, Taoist philosophy, Chinese medicine, and martial forms.

By 1931 Wan was director of the Hunan Wushu Institute. He had moved on to teach at Guangxi University by 1934 and founded the Young'an Teachers School of Physical Education in 1939. Wan went on to become a Professor of Sport at Fujian Agricultural College and remained there until his retirement in 1951.

In his lifetime, Wan authored sixteen books, including *One Zero Philosophy*, *Traditional Chinese Orthopedics*, *Zi Ran Men*, *Illustrated Shaolin Luo Han Boxing*, *Zhan Sun Fan*, *Essence of Wushu*, *Discussion of Wushu* and *24 Form Spearplay*.

Before his death Wan passed the Liu He Zi Ran Men lineage to his friend and disciple Master Hong Zhen Fu.

I started working with just a very few parts of the many sophisticated ball movements from *Ball Exercises for Health* (referred to henceforth as the Ball Book) and with the staff form from External Skills of the *Compendium*. I immediately noticed that with the ball I could actually feel clearly a bit of the "center," the elusive tanden/tantien that my instructors had constantly referred to. My dynamic balance was also improved. I realized that since one gets so completely used to one's body, its balance points are automatic and unconscious, as are its balance recovery mechanisms. The ball's weight and momentum lead the attention more clearly to the balance and recovery mechanisms and their nuances.

When working with the staff, I found that since the staff tied the hands together, thereby uniting both sides of the shoulder girdle, and that since I now had a better feeling for the center from the ball practice, I could grasp more of the concept of "whole-body" execution of technique.

The staff form proved to be an excellent introductory vehicle for studying many aspects of the ball. The various movements in the Ball Book provided an excellent foundation for enhancing martial arts techniques in such areas as jabbing, coiling, circling, weaving, cross-loading, one-sided, low to high, high to low, etc. The staff form had a great many of these movements with a really good flow and was relatively short, so I adapted the ball to the staff form and really liked the resulting combination.

Over the years I continued working with the ball and staff, elaborating and integrating them somewhat. I found this to be quite effective in providing insight into many of the problems and difficult concepts in the martial arts. The underlying principles of the ball and staff complement each other and lead to deeper levels of understanding. A lot still remains murky but some clarity has been provided regarding the center, flow, the three cardinal principles, transitions/ critical edge, internalizing, awareness, reverse breathing, etc. and a large number of "why does he do that?" or "how in hell is he able to do that?" (while practicing with or watching some particularly accomplished martial artist).

What I have done is apply the ball and staff practices to my own personal martial arts background. The insights I have gained have been very valuable and have become quite central to my martial arts understanding. Actually it seems that the more insight I gain, the more questions I find. The questions do seem to be more fundamental and focused, so hopefully that is a sign of progress. Many of my training partners have benefited as well, which is encouraging.

## My Bias toward Combat

I have a strong bias for real combat as the prime motive for martial arts training.

I suggest that this has historically been the case until comparatively recently within the culture of the individual country. The fighting came first and then, sooner or later in each martial arts culture, the other benefits were recognized and became significant.

In Japan, for example, many of the "jitsu" martial arts became "do" (way), kenjitsu to kendo, jujitsu to judo, etc., at the beginning of the Tokugawa shogunate around the time of Tokugawa Ieyasu's death, completing a vision that had been evolving for some time. See Cleary's *The Japanese Art of War* for details.

The Chou dynasty in China (1154 to about 577 BC) had a culture of chivalry that placed great weight on the character of the individual gentleman-warrior. This moral emphasis reached its height in the so-called Spring and Autumn period (766 to 577 BC) at the end of the Chou dynasty. See *The Code of the Warrior* by Rick Fields as cited in the bibliography for details.

Even Western boxing, one of the least ideological of the martial arts, has found its way into such programs as the Police Athletic League (PAL) by virtue of its ability to instill discipline and self-confidence in its participants.

A mature martial art offers its practitioners a wide range of benefits. It is extremely important that these benefits accrue to those with a benign nature. It is not true that martial arts training will make a bad person into a good person. It is much more likely to make a bad person into a more dangerous bad person.

Those whose primary training bias is for real combat choose it because real combat is really serious, with really serious consequences. Going about delivering "street justice" is not the plan. The plan is to have a group training mentality where the ultimate incentive is to have a truly serious practice where each person in the group helps others in the group achieve the broadest and deepest understanding possible for them.

## Structure of the Book

The book is divided into five main sections. The first is a Framework of ideas that presents combat-oriented ideas, concepts, and considerations that should be somewhat familiar to the reader. It will help the reader "tune in" to the more practical information in the rest of the book.

The next section on Preliminary Exercises is an introduction to the ball, getting a feel for the ball, and some basic preliminary exercises with it. This section also contains exercises from Lu Wen Wei's Ball Book, the wellspring of thought for much of this book. It also begins to apply the ideas from the framework cited above.

The third section, Forms, has the same form (kata) variously performed with the iron ball, with a wooden staff, and with empty hands. This is to compare and contrast applications of the ideas in the first two sections of the book in the three modes.

Sparring and Mobility Drills works the material from the framework of ideas, the preliminary exercises, and the forms into a coherent whole to explore the nuances and show how the information can be applied to combat. The exercises often present the difficult problems and questions of martial arts practice and suggest ways to integrate the exercises into combat solutions. The sparring material works on the practical application of the ideas and exercises to the problems of effective maneuver in combat.

Finally there is supplementary material in the Additional Practices that expands on some points in more detail. Some of it also cites ideas for training in ways that can personalize the material.

At the end are bibliographies, web sites, appendices, and an index. These have some commentary and discussion that could prove helpful.

A reasonable approach to using this book might be to read the Framework part thoroughly and then try the preliminary exercises. Reread any sections that were unclear, work through the preliminary exercises again, and then go on through to the forms and the advanced exercises. This will work very well.

If you are like me, however, you will page through the book trying things that catch your eye and then look through from the back to the front finding additional items of interest. Probably you will use the table of contents and the index a lot to rummage around amidst the contents.

In other words, you will start with the ideas that are on the cutting edge of your personal martial arts interests. Eventually you will at least sample a good deal of the ideas that pertain to your needs. This approach also works well, especially if you have good training partners to explore and work on the concepts with. Let me repeat and emphasize good training partners, good training partners, and good training partners.

## Collaborators/Contributors

This started as a personal book but, in the course of consulting with a few people about some of the material, the personal book morphed into collaboration, supported by some major contributors.

The main collaborator is my brother Curt who began martial arts practice together with me in 1957 at John Ogden's Judo and Karate school in Compton, California. He has studied Shotokan karate, Long Fist Wushu, Yang and Chen Tai Chi Chuan, and has a doctorate in classical Chinese literature. The bulk of this book's information on the internal arts comes from him.

Ron Thom, old student, friend, and fellow practitioner. I showed him the staff form back in the 1960s when I first started working on it. He has continued the practice since then and has a real feel for it. (He has developed a sword version of it.) Ron read the manuscript at several stages and provided much valuable feedback.

Tom Muzila is a very experienced all-round martial artist (fists, feet, guns, blades, clubs, military, etc.) and a good friend. The first seminar on the ball and the staff that I ever gave was held at Tom's Paramount, California, karate school in the 1980s. Tom was very much attracted to the ball practice, continued working with it over the years, and has really developed it. Check the appendix for a sample of this development. Heavyweight boxing champ Lamon Brewster, with an impressive knockout record, credits Tom's iron ball training with a significant increase in his punching power.

Joel Weinberg, old student, friend, and fellow practitioner with a very broad training background. He has a creative, multi-faceted martial arts mentality that frequently finds an overlooked angle to technique and training. I do not always agree with his new angles but he can pose excellent questions that really make you think. He is also very good at deconstructing technique application and writes about it with clarity. See the rebound discussion on page 226 for a sample of this.

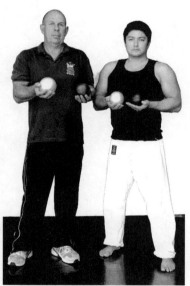

Ian O'Keefe trained intensively in Shotokan karate, boxing, Gracie jyu jitsu, Muay Thai, Jeet Kune Do, and Systema. He is one of those guys who is excellent at both the physical and the mental game in martial arts. Checking insights with him is always productive.

Dave and Chris Shaver. They are two very good friends and fellow practitioners for many years. They have extensive backgrounds in Shotokan karate, boxing, and practical applied combat. Dave studied fencing with a European old-timer who was a for-real dueling specialist (dagger in the back hand and other realistic deadly stuff). The biomechanics Dave learned

**Figure 3: Thanks to Dave Shaver and Esteban Ramiriz for their help with the pictures in this book.**

from fencing have benefited his training partners greatly. Studying Chris's intuitive body sense and targeting system is always profitable and Dave's long-ago observations on the initiation role of the hands and feet were inspired. I have to pay close attention while speaking with them. They throw out really good insights offhandedly and keep going. Listen or miss them.

Finally, a thousand thanks to my training partners in the martial arts class at the South Bay Dojo in Hawthorne, California: Juan, Esteban, Mark, Randy, Bob, and Collie, all led by Dave and Chris. Their insightful questions and dedicated efforts truly helped focus my thought and shape this book.

# 2. Framework

When I began experimenting with the iron ball back in the 1960s, I tried to apply it to everything. Timewise this was totally impractical and yielded very mixed results. Gradually a few basic themes emerged, which were giving me much better insights. I found that nearly all the goals and objectives of my martial arts practice could be clearly referenced to these basic themes. This resulted in a framework for practice that was easy to effectively hang almost any martial arts idea I encountered on.

There are three primary concepts that I want to emphasize: structure, flow, and maneuver. Each of them is a Big Deal. You will find parts that you already understand and some that might seem like different interpretations, or perhaps things you consider not very important. Just give the framework and the ball a chance. This format worked very well for those I practiced with and the experiences of those who developed a good familiarity with the ball have been very positive. Indeed, fresh viewpoints in the martial arts can yield true breakthroughs in understanding. I'm including them here because I find them valuable for most aspects of the practice. Some things are best understood with one model; some are best understood with another. Here is a brief introduction to the three primary concepts.

**Structure:** You frequently hear of someone having good "form." This is too suggestive of just outward appearance. I prefer to use the term "structure," which denotes both internal and external characteristics. This is the combat structure of the body, which differs somewhat from the normal body in posture and use. Structure includes three biomechanical systems: centers (perhaps as many as four), integrative action paths/energy channels (mother line and centerline), and initiators (feet, hands, and intent/mind). Somewhat advanced structural concerns deal with internalizing concepts such as core energy transference, chi, energetics understanding, etc.

**Flow:** The dynamic physical and mental fluidity of combat. Appropriately maneuvering a well-integrated structure in combat without any fatal lapses requires a good, constant flow. This is effectively realized by close attention to nuances of such things as breathing, integrating mind and body, center management, critical edge maintenance, rebound management, chi management, etc.

**Maneuver:** Basically these are mobility concepts and considerations essential to effective use of the structure when executing techniques in combat. Examples would be centering, effective critical edge and transition usage, good flow, opponent connection, "room" awareness, etc.

There is a great deal of overlap in flow and maneuver but there are also differences. I feel that making the distinction is quite useful.

I think that good flow, for the most part, is the ability to move an effective combat structure seamlessly through combat maneuvers without any mental or physical lapses. A thorough integration of the three body-system dynamics is a must. Flow is studied much of the time by monitoring foot plant, the centers, breathing, balance points, transitions, critical edge function, etc. while performing exercises. A lot of this is performed with an internal self-monitoring mindset. Errors are noted and corrected. Frequently, flow errors stem from problems with structure so you would circle back to deal with the structural problem. Although you are not at that point practicing "real" combat, this is a totally necessary part of the learning process, which then progresses into a more realistic combat-oriented version of the concept.

The ball practice can really enhance insight into the nuances of structure and flow. I find myself frequently coming back to look at the more fundamental ball and staff drills for additional insight and clues for variations that might prove productive.

Maneuver has a strategic component that is always present. It is a very practical vision of the application of an effective mental and physical combat structure against an opponent. As such, a majority of the study of maneuver involves visualized opponents, opponent substitutes, or real training partners. There is much more of an external mind set. Errors are usually obvious, sometimes painfully so. Correction of errors frequently requires circling back to further inquiry of structure and flow.

The very best combat drills bridge the requirements of structure, flow, and maneuver without leaving any reality gaps.

**Critical edge** is a concept that spans the three primary concepts of structure, flow, and maneuver, varying in consideration according to the context. I feel that it is a particularly important concept (a Big Deal) and should be a major benchmark in martial arts practice. I found that the ball practice was an excellent training aid for enhancing critical edge "feel" and exploring its nuances.

The critical edge is your mental and physical orientation against your opponent. Being on the critical edge means maintenance of that physical and mental posture whereby the slightest physical or mental gesture can impel/release you against your opponent. In a certain sense, because you are so finely balanced, even while standing still you are in motion. Think of the person balanced on a high wire. There are constant subtle adjustments.

Do you remember seeing an opening while sparring that was right there but you were just not ready to attack? Or being caught flat-footed by an attack that you saw coming a mile away but you got nailed anyway? If you had been mentally and physically on the critical edge, your chances for a positive outcome would have been much improved. Drills, fundamentals, forms, and sparring that focus on developing your ability to feel the critical edge are certainly among the most important you can practice.

To find and maintain the critical edge in a static state is not so hard to do. However, to remain always on the critical edge while maneuvering in front of a dangerous person is quite difficult. The dynamic critical edge is the real challenge. Training with the ball adds enough destabilizing resistance to reveal even minor deviations from the ideal.

A note on the phrase "critical edge": I formerly used the inclusive term "transition point" to describe this more specific concept. After training in Jeet Kune Do with Pat Strong I feel that his term, critical edge, is more selective, descriptive, and nuanced in regard to combat-opponent orientation.

There is of course much, much more to martial arts practice than the above but these are very important and the ball practice is particularly suited to their study and to other related material.

## *How to Use This Framework*

The ideas to be presented all fit into one or more of the three primary concepts above. No doubt the material cited in the definitions of the three concepts above could be organized in other ways, but because of the nature of the ball practice and what I feel are its particular virtues, this is the best I have found.

First the ideas are presented, followed by some definition and discussion of the ideas.

Next are preliminary exercises to "sample" the ideas followed by some forms to contrast the ball, weapon, and empty hand versions of the ideas. The forms are triple benchmarks for your understanding of the ideas. As your understanding evolves, form performance is adjusted and correspondingly evolves.

Then there are sparring/drill type exercises using the ball, staff, empty hands, and equipment to work on applying the ideas in a combat-type situation; basically maneuver practices to develop effective maneuver technique but also designed to explore and test the relative lethality of your technique. This is where true understanding and integration of the concepts is developed. Hopefully good training partners to provide honest tests and good feedback will be available for this.

### Visualizing Aids

Quite a few of the ideas are presented in the form of visualizing aids. These are mental tools used to help the learning process. Some are engineering-like biomechanical visualizations, some the intuitive energetics type, some are a mixture of the two. Examples would be the center (or centers), chi, the mother line, etc.

These visualizing aids permeate the Asian martial arts and can be very effective in enhancing technique. I feel that everyone should at least try to use them because they can really jumpstart your technique, but be careful that they do not become an end in themselves. Do not habitually let the visualizations come between you and your opponents. Closely monitoring your center visualization while in range of your opponent in a fairly serious match is unrealistic. (I cite this example because of personal experiences involving pain.) The idea is to use the visualizations until they become a natural, ingrained part of your technique and then move them back out of your consciousness.

## Objectives/Goals

Within the framework there are some very desirable objectives or goals to keep in mind while you practice. Some of these should be carefully noted. A prime example is internalizing your technique application (withdrawing side understanding, the "empty arm" punch, core energy transference, and rebound management). A good understanding of the internalizing concept and its nuances will greatly enhance the effectiveness of your martial arts practice. NOTE: by internalizing I do not refer to the internal/energetic arts; I mean the "gateway" process of refining and enhancing technique application, which is discussed throughout this text. Other important goals and objectives are breath management, a defensive and offensive ability to "read" your opponent, educated feet, injury avoidance, etc.

I will cite one example of injury avoidance because I feel it is a very important one.

**Negative maintenance** is continuing to practice superfluous, questionable, erroneous, or destructive techniques because they "feel right" or are considered traditional. Surprisingly, many people find reasons to do so. It's not a good idea however and leads to a lot of avoidable injuries, some of them serious.

I feel that using some of the exercises in this book could help you avoid many of these problems. The added weight of the ball will refine your balance points and alter your normal movement patterns. You will be able to look at your movements and techniques from another perspective and discover previously unnoticed destructive stresses.

It has helped me tremendously. I credit the ball and staff practice with preserving my marginal low back condition and with keeping my hip joints from continuing down the road to replacement by fine-tuning my biomechanics.

# Structure

This is the first part of the framework for this book. Any physical art such as dance, gymnastics, yoga, football, etc. has requirements that result in specific optimum or at least highly desirable models of the body as it is to be used. The martial arts are no exception. The wide variety of martial arts leads to many models, but since we are talking about combat and since the whole body is a weapon, there are several universal elements that apply to them all.

## Four Models

When I consider structure, I have four models I use to describe what is there. The various models deserve serious attention and experimentation.

The first is an external, internal, or blended type practitioner who uses a single-center visualization.

The second is an internal visualization from Lu Wen Wei, which has four centers. (Obviously external martial artists can also use multiple-center visualizations.) This is a minority opinion since the single tantien (center) model is currently the most prevalent.

The third model is the anatomical/kinesiological three activity centers of Ida Rolf, who is famous for her understanding about how structural integration contributes to health and well-being.

The fourth is a biomechanical function approach using three body systems as they directly apply to martial arts. These are the locomotor/transport/energy system, the manipulative member system, and the cognitive processor/sense organ cluster system. This last is a useful framework for comparing and exploring the nuances of the various models.

All of these models have similar, but not identical, descriptions of the systems/centers involved in structure and how they are organized to integrate and work together. Each has its place in thinking about the best way to use the body for effective execution of martial arts techniques.

The various versions of the centers — mother line with extensions, centerline, and chi applications — are all visualizations. Ida Rolf's model is an anatomical/kinesiological description of biomechanical action in critical activity areas of the human body. The biomechanical model describes the anatomical/kinesiological actions of the visualization on a systemic and whole-body basis. This information can lead to an extremely valuable understanding of the physical basis of martial art training.

The center (or centers) is definitely a Big Deal. There are many definitions and descriptions and most work very well indeed for the individual style. Usually the centers are indicated by a single point, although it is obvious that they are larger in activity. The center is a major visualizing aid.

For most Asian-style martial artists the two major overall categories of the martial arts are the external/biomechanical or the internal/energy models. In both models the "center" is a Big Deal. With the external model the "center" is the major intersection and focus of the biomechanical forces used in executing techniques. With the internal model the center is the intersection and reservoir of the energy forces used in executing techniques. The blended internal/external Asian styles get to work with both points of view.

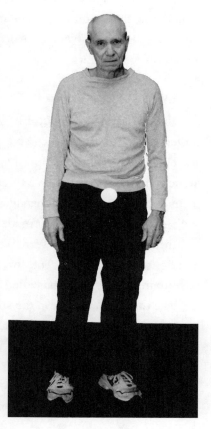

**Figure 4: THE center point in the tantien.**

### THE Center

There is one primary center that most martial artists recognize. One could call it THE center. Almost all Asian arts will give a general location of THE center in the lower abdomen. Western arts such as boxing do not have a defined concept for the center but clearly use the hips and mother line in instruction, and most effectively indeed in application.

I certainly agree with the existence of THE center, but I have found that visualizing three (or four) centers adds considerably to my understanding of technique. Lu Wen Wei, Ida Rolf, and the biomechanical model all use models with multiples centers.

### Lu Wen Wei's Centers

Hsing Yi boxing, which Lu Wen Wei's father practiced, also visualizes three centers. They are located close to, but are not identical with, Lu's centers. They are considered locations for the generation, storage, and transmission of chi. Some other internal arts have three centers — you can find many on the web that seem to be devoted to chi management almost exclusively.

Here is the Lu Wen Wei model I found to be so valuable.

In his Ball Book Lu Wen Wei says there are four tantiens (centers): lower, middle, and two upper. The lower is below the navel, which is the traditional positioning, what might be called THE center.

The middle center is on the spine at jaiji zhong huang tantien (middle yellow, governing vessel 10 on the acupuncture charts, which is between the 6th and 7th thoracic spinous processes).

One upper tantien is between the eyes. Lu Wen Wei then goes on to say that

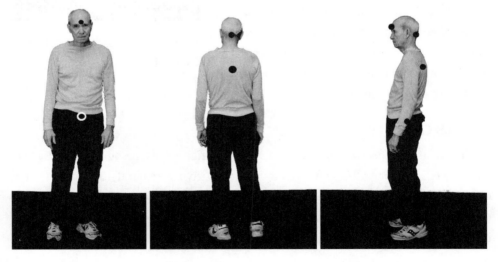

**Figure 5: Lu Wen Wei's four centers, front, back, and side view.**

there is yet another center at the back of the skull at the join of the neck (governing vessel 16 on the acupuncture chart, and which is the sub-occipital triangle/cranial-cervical junction anatomically). Significantly, the sub-occipital triangle is a muscle complex that together with the pre-vertebral muscles integrates with the eye and ear balance mechanisms for orienting to the horizon and for making the fine cranial adjustments necessary to help the eyes follow erratically flying objects such as mosquitoes or fists.

Lu Wen Wei's upper center between the eyes and the lower center are generally in accord with the three-center systems, but his middle center and his additional center at the cranial join of the neck are quite different. I speculate that this is because he replaced Tai Chi techniques with ball movements based on the ball system of his father. It may not have been his original intent, but the ball likely educated him to a middle center and an additional upper center required for effective fighting. He ended up with a middle center and an additional upper center located more for combat than for chi management. This is where external and internal combat-oriented practitioners will start paying serious attention. There is more on this later in the chapter.

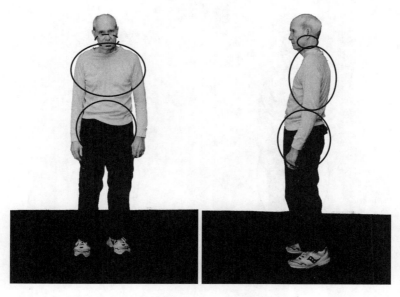

**Figure 6: Ida Rolf's activity centers, front view and side view.**

### Ida Rolf's Centers

The four tantiens of Lu Wen Wei accord nicely with the therapeutic "three activity centers" in the anatomical/kinesiological body model of Ida Rolf. Repairing and integrating the pelvic girdle, shoulder girdle, and the cranial-cervical junction (precisely Lu Wen Wei's fourth center) is a major part of Rolfing therapy. Ida Rolf's preferred term for the therapy named for her was structural integration. Those who have been Rolfed can attest to the improvement in body movement they experience. After Rolfing the "centers" work the way they are meant to.

Ida Rolf was an intuitive genius who "saw" how the body best needed to work. She and Lu Wen Wei would have seen eye to eye. Her books discuss the vertical thrust and other Rolfing concepts that can easily apply to martial arts. In particular her book, *Rolfing*, depicts the centers and their musculature so well and discusses their action so clearly that their concordance with Lu Wen Wei's centers is obvious. Also obvious is their value in bringing understanding to such important problems as center integration, which is discussed below.

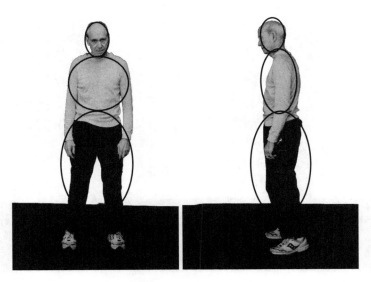

**Figure 7: System biomechanics centers, front view and side view.**

## Biomechanical Systems

This biomechanical model divides the body into the locomo-tor/transport/energy (in the pelvic region), manipulative member (related to the shoulder girdle), and the sense organ cluster/cognitive processor/cranial-cervical junction systems. Looking at the body this way provides an additional biomechanical way to think about understanding how these particular action "centers" function and how to integrate body movement for effective technique. A lot of anatomical and kinesiological function will be glossed over because this model is to provide insight into the specific visualized centers, not a comprehensive analysis of martial arts biomechanics. Such an analysis would be a massive project.

## Centers and Martial Arts

Ultimately these four models are complementary and all are well worth exploring. This makes a great deal of sense on many levels. By considering the objectives and difficult problems of martial arts practice in terms of the three body systems and Ida Rolf's three activity centers, the external arts are covered. The single tantien model and Lu Wen Wei's four tantiens concept does the same for the internal arts. Obviously the external arts can and do use the single and multi-tantien visualizations. This multi-pronged approach offers better chances of success with the internalizing core energy transfer, empty arm punch techniques, and other frequently vexing martial arts goals.

Most Asian martial arts talk about one center, the tanden/tantien somewhere in the pelvic region. The center is a crucial element of effective technique. While I believe that this may be the most important center, visualizing and working with the other centers described by Lu Wen Wei, Ida Rolf, and system biome-chanics added a great deal more to my martial arts understanding.

Obviously the systems/centers of the martial arts body must be well inte-grated for effective structure and its utilization. These centers are located and "centered" on the mother line. (The mother line is discussed further on page 34). When considering the centers and the mother line, looking at them from the perspectives of Lu Wen Wei, Ida Rolf, and system biomechanics is productive. The multi-pronged approach applies here as well. Studying the structure and the critical issue of integration of the body from multiple perspectives can provide good insights and a broader understanding of the exercises in the book.

### Lower Center: The locomotor/transport/ energy system

Lu Wen Wei puts the lower center below the navel, which is the traditional positioning that most martial artists recognize. In the rest of the book I will be calling it THE center. Understanding and insights related to the lower center would, for the most part, also apply to Lu Wen Wei's middle center.

Ida Rolf calls this the pelvic girdle activity center. For Rolfers this is a very Big Deal, correcting structural and postural imbalances in the pelvic girdle is a major part of their very successful therapy. Successful pelvic girdle Rolfing therapy starts with the feet.

From a biomechanical system perspective the first center consists of the feet, legs, and pelvic girdle.

For me, the locus of THE center is just in front of the spinal column at about the level of the fifth lumbar vertebra. I believe this because this area seems to be the intersection of biomechanical forces that result in effective whole-body movement. After working with the ball for a time it seemed that this specific area was the most effective at moving the ball and the body in all planes of motion.

The center is active, not a static point or pivot. That sense of a dynamic, controlling intersection of forces transferred quite easily to all movement and I did feel that the effectiveness of my technique was markedly enhanced. During this time my structure, foot position (and appreciation of the major significance of

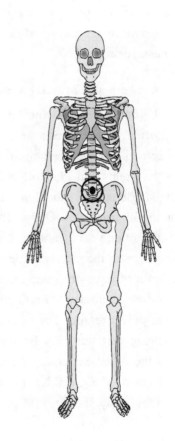

**Figure 8: THE Center location just in front of the spinal column about the level of the fifth lumbar vertebra.**

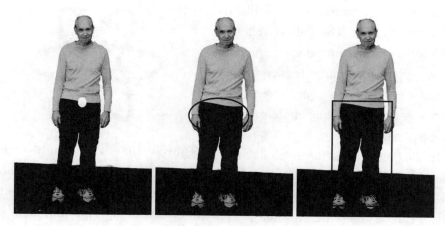

**Figure 9: The lower center: Lu Wen Wei's lower center (THE Center), Ida Rolf's center, and the biomechanical system center.**

the foot), stepping, and movement mechanics changed considerably and for the better. Some of the changes occurred without my being aware of them at first. The ball practice corrected problems I had not been aware of. This is my own perception, based on my individual use of structure and techniques.

Because this center is so important, considering the views of some other practitioners about this center before going on to look at the other centers will provide for a broader view of it.

The Japanese word for center is tanden (sometimes "hips" in translation). Master Egami, during his 1973 visit to our Shotokan group in Los Angeles, made the statement that "hips includes knees" which was an epiphany for us.

The Chinese term is tantien. Wang Shu Jin in his Bagua book calls it the center of bodily gravity and weightlessness; which is a provocative juxtaposition of terms.

According to my brother Curt, internal stylists fill (or visualize filling) the tantien with a chi ball which needs to be sealed on the bottom and at the top. On the bottom this is accomplished by sealing the hui yin cavity, lightly tightening the anus to do so. At the top, the sealing is accomplished by the relaxing and sinking of the diaphragm. The chi ball expands (and contracts?) in all directions encountering the seals until it fills (or packs) the tantien. The ball is felt as a multi-vector dynamically spinning/ rotating sphere that transmits energy.

Some visualize a continually expanding and contracting circle/sphere of connected parts.

In another model, the rotation of the abdominal ball in an infinite number of ways transmits energy to the rest of the body. (This is the visualization I have chosen.) Tantien rotation can operate as a basic energy but typically generates spirals that permeate the body, though some spirals can be accomplished without tantien rotation. The goal is for any slight movement in any one part of the body to generate complementary movement throughout the whole body. Obviously there are a lot of details to work on.

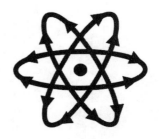

**Figure 10: The multi-vector, rotating ball, shown here without most of its vectors and the center point exposed. This model works for Lu Wen Wei's lower, middle, and upper cranial/ cervical junction centers. It also works for the internal stylists' multi-vector spinning/rotating sphere that transmits energy, as well as the infinite-way rotating abdominal ball that transmits energy to the rest of the body.**

External stylists feel THE center as a power and activity intersection in about the same location. For many this center is large with layers like an onion. It includes the knees and shoulder girdle.

The multi-vector, infinite-way, rotating-ball center visualizations can work very well for external stylists. This was an early discovery for me in my ball practice. Up to that point I had a basically horizontal-plane hip rotating model of the center, raising and lowering the plane but not taking full advantage of the inherent versatility of the pelvic girdle.

- - -

The locomotor/transport/energy system of the lower center is anchored in the feet. In terms of structure, the feet are definitely worth careful consideration.

Effective use of the feet is a major goal in the martial arts. Like the hands, the feet are very versatile parts of the human anatomy, capable of a broad range of conscious and unconscious use. Functionally the feet are somewhat like an automotive suspension system with springs and shock absorbers. They even include a power train and a steering system and play a major role in initiating system usage.

The question commonly posed with regard to foot plant concerns the best contact with the ground for the foot. Western boxers typically maneuver on the balls of their feet, going more flatfooted for power punches. Some traditional Asian arts are rather flatfooted and can include the role of the heel in maneuver. My original art is one of those. Some give several specific locations for foot plant points (e.g., William C.C. Chen's three nails). The study of foot plant is of extreme importance and one that should be pursued both within and without the training hall.

Ball practice can really help develop a feeling for foot action and test your understanding of it. For example, visualizing your feet moving the ball in the exercises can really accelerate development of effectively educated feet. Training

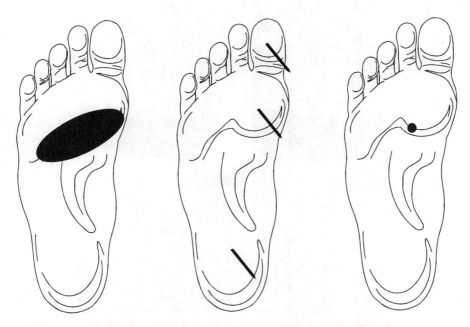

**Figure 11: Foot plants: Western boxing, the location of William C.C. Chen's three nails, and the bubbling well.**

on a variety of surfaces will also enhance foot education.

The bubbling well is a plant point on the foot common in Tai Chi Chuan, and is one of several effective versions of foot plant points available for managing use of the feet in the martial arts. Interestingly, for acupuncturists it is point Yong Quan, K-1 on the kidney (energy) meridian. They also call it the corpse revival point. It is located in the arches just back of the ball of the foot between the first and second metatarsal bones.

Personally I have come to like this plant point a lot because it gives me more spring energy and ready maneuverability than other versions I have tried.

### Middle Center: The manipulative members system

Lu Wen Wei's middle center is on the spine at jaiji zhong huang tantien (between the sixth and seventh thoracic spinous processes). The location is not intuitive — one might think the location would be directly between the shoulder

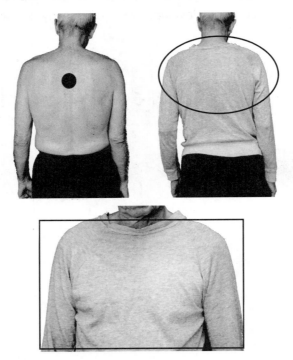

**Figure 12: The middle center: Lu Wen Wei's middle center, Ida Rolf's shoulder girdle activity center, and the middle biomechanical system center.**

sockets of the arms. The advantage of his position is that the common destabilizing problems of tension and power going up are much easier to manage, and integrating with the upper center is much more natural. Also, the shoulders feel like they are more readily available as a mobile part of the arms. It's a mistake to lock the shoulder to the torso for almost all techniques because this tends to create local power and inhibits versatility and flow of arm movement.

This center is Ida Rolf's shoulder girdle activity center. The "activities" she

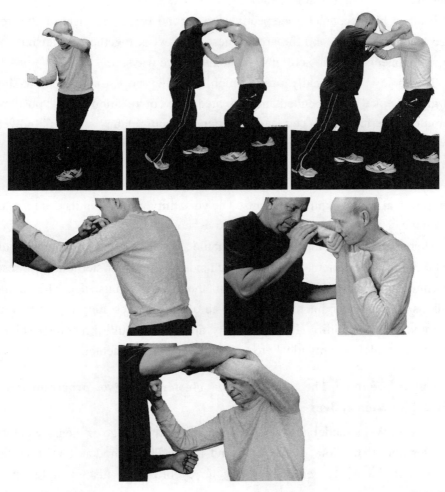

**Figure 13: The mobility of the shoulder girdle, as shown in applications.**

refers to are virtually all muscular. Muscle imbalances here create real problems with local power, balance, flow, and correct biomechanics. Incorrect biomechanics frequently leads to injuries and can markedly affect power output. Rolfing therapy is directed to correcting such imbalances. I can attest to this from personal experience. My Rolfer, Steve Bankes, corrected a host of imbalances resulting from my broken neck, restoring me to a near normal posture. There was an amazing improvement. Also, as a health consultant, some of the work I do is Rolfing type and many of my clients, quite a few of them martial artists, have benefited a lot from it, Danny Inosanto, for an example.

From a biomechanical perspective the second center consists of the upper torso, shoulder girdle, and the arms. These parts work together to transmit force to the opponents in various offensive and defensive ways.

The torso is functionally a rather mobile springy post from which the shoulder girdle "yoke" is suspended and activated. The composition of the "post" with its multiple vertebrae, rib cage, and surrounding musculature ensures a powerful mobility for the spirals, coiling and uncoiling, compressions and expansions, etc. of martial arts technique.

The shoulder girdle, including arms and hands, is statistically the most common physical contact with opponents. The versatility inherent in its design allows for a wide choice of offensive and defensive "contacts."

There is just one joint in the torso/shoulder girdle connection, the clavicular-manubrial joint (two actually, one on each side of the upper sternum); the rest of the connections of the shoulder girdle to the torso are muscular. The shoulder girdle is suspended and activated by a web of muscles resulting in a very versatile movement capability. This versatility allows the multi-directional spinning ball center model to apply nicely to Lu Wen Wei's middle center.

**Upper Center: The sense organ cluster/cognitive processor/cranial cervical junction system**

Lu Wen Wei's model has two centers here (on the bridge of the nose between the eyes and at the join of the head and neck). Other models that have three centers put the upper center between the eyebrows or just up a bit on the forehead.

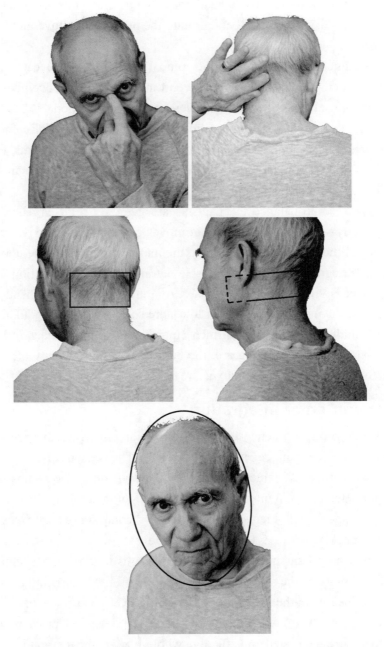

**Figure 14: The upper center: Lu Wen Wei's two upper centers, Ida Rolf's cranial-cervical junction, and the upper biomechanical system center.**

Ida Rolf terms Lu Wen Wei's head-neck join as the cranial-cervical junction activity center. Basically it is a band around the neck, a bit above and below the cranial-cervical junction.

Biomechanically this includes the mind (brain), eyes, the ears with their attendant balancing mechanisms, which coordinate with the suboccipital triangle/ pre-vertebral muscle complex, and the eyes for body orientation.

The cognitive processor — the mind — leads all systems with intent, thereby directing action and energy. The sense organ cluster senses opponents, the room, and the self in relation to them. The cranial-cervical junction is an effective orientation/targeting enabler.

Of course, some balance mechanisms are ganglion reflexes, some sensory inputs are body-wide, and some combat moves can become reflexive, but intent has developed those reflexes and refined the moves. Intent from the upper center initiates the integration process of muscle entrainment, joint selection, etc. Integration proceeds virtually simultaneously from the head, feet, and hands through all centers via the mother line in order to ensure correct sequencing. (This may be effectively studied in slow motion.) The more combat appropriate and comprehensive your drills and sparring are, the better; checking as many of the arts as possible for ideas is really productive.

## System/Center Integration

Considering one's practice of drills, forms, and sparring in terms of these systems and centers can be extremely helpful. The various divisions provide either an energetic or a biomechanically logical division of the combat structure and the problems found in integrating and applying it in combat.

So many specific problems, such as the very common one of excessive tension in the neck that raises the shoulders and can disturb the structure of the whole body, are system-specific. This tension results in local power inhibition of the desired fluidity of the system. According to Ida Rolf, integration of the pelvic girdle/center begins in the feet, for another example. A clear understanding of the entire system involved can eliminate both seen and unseen problems, thereby leading to a more integrated and effective whole-body combat structure.

By integration I mean uniting and managing the locomotor/transport/energy unit together with the manipulative members by and with the sense organ cluster/cognitive processor/cranial-cervical junction in the most efficient way. Ideally

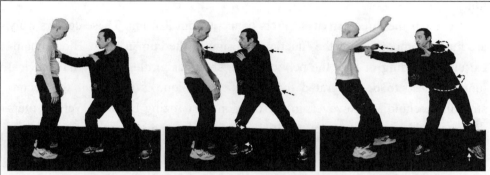

**Figure 15: Bruce Lee's one-inch punch demonstrated by Joel Weinberg as an example of integrating all the body systems. This sequence works quite clearly because this is a very simple move in spite of its complex internal integration of the centers. One can see that this is an effective stand-alone technique but could also be the end point of a stepping or body-shifting maneuver.**

**In picture one a neutral body posture is shown. In picture two there is an initial forward impulse from hip and middle center with a simultaneous pulse from the feet that drives the lower center in a bit. The weight shifts forward, yielding a strong penetrating action accompanied by a powerful arm impulse. In picture three the lower center simultaneously rotates around the mother line with the weight shift augmenting the middle center thrust with the back leg providing much of this force. This is a result of the rear leg pivoting on the ball of the foot and forcing the heel and leg upward with a powerful foot extension. In picture three we also see the completion of the sequence where the sudden integrated centers impulse ebbs but the mental focus on the target remains. Obviously intent from the upper center initiated and guided these actions.**

**This is a typical expansive application of the empty arm principle discussed on page 63.**

the mind and body is one unit while executing techniques. The mind moves and all that can contribute does, all that cannot goes along without inhibition.

The problem is identifying the contributors and the inhibitors within a given technique. Separating the body into three systems aids the process of identification.

Consider the three-activity-centers concept from Rolfing. These centers truly are major components of the functional design of the human body. Biomechanical understanding of how the pelvic girdle, shoulder girdle, and cranial-cervical junction need to be integrated for effective technique is important for deconstructing technique. However, in my opinion, visualizing Lu Wen Wei's centers concept is more useful, at least initially when I am trying to manage the many problems I find when trying to develop the most effective structure.

## Mother Line

The term "mother line" is used because there were differences in the center-line route (vertical axis) from various sources. The action and energetic routes from the Hsing Yi and Mantak Chia information were in basic agreement regarding the spinal column route as shown in Figure 16. Since a very common centerline route from external and internal schools extends from a point between the feet through the perineum to the top of the head, I chose to differentiate these two differing routes by choosing another name for the spinal route, which I borrowed from Pat Strong.

In addition, mother line extension through the limbs to the hands and feet and around the head as shown so well in the Mantak Chia illustration (Figure 17) seemed right intuitively. Intuition was definitely reinforced by good progress with the ball work using this model.

In Lu Wen Wei's approach, two of the multiple centers are located on the mother line. The mother line from THE center passes up through the middle center to and into the upper centers. This is an important element of his multiple center visualization. Linking and integrating the centers largely begins with intent from the upper center when action is indicated. Or to state it another way, the cognitive processor, probably informed by the sense organ cluster, directs the locomotor/transport/energy system and/or the manipulative member system to

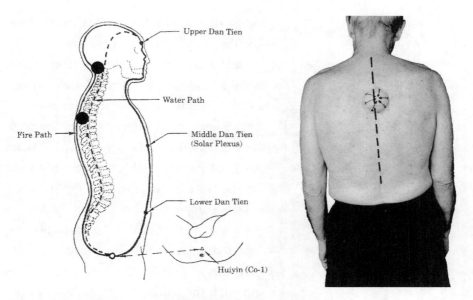

**Figure 16: Huiyin cavity illustration from *Hsing Yi Chuan* (p. 51). The spinal part of the mother line with two of Lu's centers shown by the dots (●). The back view shows the location of the paths.[2]**

take (hopefully) appropriate action. Of the various visualizations I have tried, this mother line model feels the most natural and is the easiest to lapse into the background yet still be present.

The center/centering/mother line/etc. concepts are vehicles for understanding how to achieve the integration objective in an intuitive way rather than bogging down in a mass of anatomical and kinesiological detail. I feel that it is quicker and easier for most people to take the intuitive visualized step and then subsequently do the biomechanical assessments to see how they got there. Obviously, understanding both approaches would be better but not strictly necessary if you are making good progress.

In the internal model the mother line is the term used to describe the main energetic channels between the centers and, for some, to trace additional ener-

---

[2] From *Hsing Yi Chuan, Theory and Applications,* Liang Shou-Yu and Yang Jwing-Ming, published by YMAA Publication Center, Inc, 1990. Reproduced with permission of YMAA Publication Center, Inc.

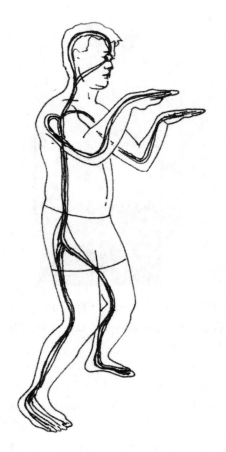

**Figure 17: Mother line visualization from Mantak Chia.**

getic flow routes. It extends from the base of the body up through the core of THE center and up the spinal column to the top of the head. The exact route varies somewhat depending on who you talk to.

Some practitioners also visualize extensions down the legs to the ground and out the arms. This feels exactly right to me since it works equally well with the external approach.

Although Mantak Chia does not use the term mother line, his illustrated route for energy flow in the torso and neck is through the spinal column. He states (on page 222) that the very center of our physical structure is the spine and its foundation, the pelvis. He notes the sacral and cranial pumps for cerebrospinal fluid which accord well with the Hsing Yi water line. Encased within the spine and cranium is the central nervous system, the center of our conscious life. Thus structural health of the spine is the foundation for the structural and energetic health of the body.

Note the cranial route of Mantak Chia's full mother line with extensions. It passes around the top of the cranium down to Lu Wen Wei's upper center and then continues right past the bottom of the brain to reconnect with the cervical mother line. Since the spinal route of the mother line is neurological, ending/originating in the brain, the cranial nerves that originate in the bottom of the brain and have the balance, sight, hearing, etc. functions really could be considered part of the mother line or at least mother line extensions.

After working with Lu Wen Wei's multiple centers concept, I have come to feel that the mother line basically runs with the curves of the spinal column. Since the spinal column is functionally a spring, an inner core energy center, and a major neurological unit (spinal cord), among its various functions, it provides a resilient, dynamically powered interface for the four centers. This would be true if you are thinking either biomechanically or energetically. It can be a major energetics channel or a biomechanical central power device. The mother line is an extremely effective visualizing aid for developing "whole-body" technique, maintaining an effectively integrated structure, fluid, effective expansion and contraction, and internalizing techniques (core energy transfer, the empty arm punch, etc.). The mother line and the centerline are two separate visualizations. As far as I can tell, the centerline visualization is functionally in direct conflict with Lu's visualization.

## Centerline

The centerline is similar to the mother line in its intended usage. As shown in the illustration, it extends from a point between the feet through the perineum to the top of the head. It seems to be a straight line through the vertical axis of the body mass and not totally oriented to internal body structure.

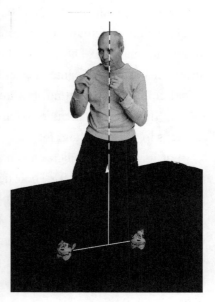

I have had no success whatsoever trying to visualize simultaneously the centerline and the mother line, as I understand it. It seems to be an either-or proposition in execution.

I have tried working with this centerline in flow and maneuver and found that it worked well with the outer core muscles, in particular the external oblique, internal oblique, and the transverse abdominus (these muscles also work very well with the mother line). I had more problems when trying to visualize and integrate Lu Wen Wei's centers with a

**Figure 18: The centerline.**

centerline visualization than with a spinal-column-oriented mother line. In addition I felt a bit constrained somehow and my torso felt less supple. Until I get some good information on centerline definition and applications from a knowledgeable person, I am using the mother line instead.

An excellent example of system integration and a good look at internalizing of technique is shown in the Bobby Taboada shadow form lesson in tape 8 of his instructional series on the Balintawak Escrima Cuentada system.

The students accompanying Mr. Taboada in the instructional form breakdown are fairly advanced. The body systems are well integrated and the strikes occur as one, with a simultaneous whole-body movement from the feet to the hands. The students execute rather extreme willowy "dragon body" movements that are obviously very effective.

When Mr. Taboada executes these techniques, they are very subtle, simultaneous, integrated whole-body movements that are obviously very effective. The dragon has been internalized.

## Using the Center Models

I have come to feel that the lower tantien (single center model) is the center of THE center and that the whole center is actually quite substantial physically, and quite nuanced. The mother line, for example, is an extension of the center basically running up the spinal column transmitting its force or energy. Some mother line models include extensions out the arms and legs to the hands and feet, as shown in Figure 17.

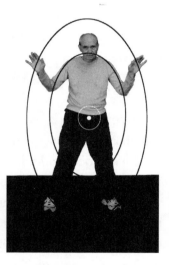

For many practitioners the center has layers, like an onion. (See Figure 19.) Their descriptions indicate that the larger center, including the knees and shoulder girdle, is always used but this use becomes unconscious with familiarity. Finally just the tantien ball/intersection is conscious and then even that can become unconscious and automatic. I live for the day!

**Figure 19: The center's layers surrounding THE center point.**

I used the layered single-center model for quite a while. It worked very well, using the feet to initiate bottom of the tantien knee action, which acted simultaneously through the tantien intersection to move the ball-manipulating top of the tantien shoulder girdle. I was by then visualizing THE center as a multi-vector rotating sphere. Nuances of ball manipulation led to visualizing a spring-like mother line extension up the spinal column.

The final single-center visualization I ended up with is the multi-vector rotating sphere onion, with mother line extensions down the legs to the toes and up the spinal column to the shoulder girdle and head with extensions out the arms to the fingers.

In working with Lu Wen Wei's four centers model (Figure 20) and while focusing on integrating the upper centers, I found very early on that empty hand drills and some boxing combinations were improved markedly. Weapons work also improved a lot. The middle center visualization of the shoulder girdle, after a frequently frustrating time, made weapons feel nearly as familiar as empty hands. This was especially effective after incorporating the multi-vector rotating ball visualization to the middle center.

Feeling that the hands and feet were initiating the middle center rotating ball without visualizing the lower center was the first step. This was particularly

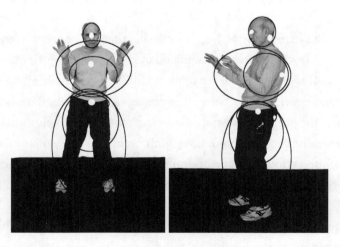

**Figure 20: The multi-center model showing the onion layers.**

noticeable when going back and forth between the ball and a striking bag. The rotating ball visualization provided readier speed and noticeably more force to upper body techniques. It also felt more natural when working on internalizing. Adding this more familiar lower center multi-vector rotating ball visualization to the middle center has really benefited me in both self-practice and sparring. The iron ball is a type of lie detector biomechanically. I have been working with it for a long time and, when I got the middle center going really well with the ball, I knew I was on the right track. I learned a lot by working selected centers independently to find each center's problems and their nuances.

Getting the upper and middle centers going together with the hands and feet followed seamlessly — naturally, since the mother line links all centers.

Working to visualize all four centers simultaneously was fairly easy while practicing maneuvering without an additional specific purpose; but when trying to also work on something like internalizing, which has its own complexities, I tended to lose a center. Adding a bit of emphasis to foot-knee action helped solve the problem. Actually, progressing from visualizing to consistently and effectively using all four centers went more smoothly and quickly than I anticipated when I started.

After my body has fully absorbed and integrated it all, I may return to the single center model. (Possible, but not likely.) However, I am sure that if I do so, I will have benefited very much from the broad exploration of the multiple-center concept.

I feel that the main thing to keep in mind is that the concept of the center is a proven tool that leads to advanced understanding. Becoming fixated on a single vision of the tool without exploring other possible visions is limiting the range of your understanding. In this, as with other concepts, a large toolbox is better.

Obviously the central question about center model exploration is whether there is a generally superior model. As with breathing and some other concepts, the models of the various styles work quite well. Satisfaction with the concepts of one's own style, however, should not preclude investigation of the thought and technique of others.

The center concept really is a Big Deal, crucial to effective combat technique usage; unexamined "brand loyalty" would be a serious mistake here.

## Combat Posture

Ideal normal posture for combat is something like the military posture except that the military people "brace" into it rather than use a relaxed expansion into the normal posture.

In the combat posture the chest is softened and the back widens. This releases and mobilizes the shoulders. The pelvis tucks up somewhat, straightening out the lower back curve a bit. (There are several ways the various arts adjust the lower back conformation: tuck the pelvis in, let the sacrum hang, etc.) The buttocks

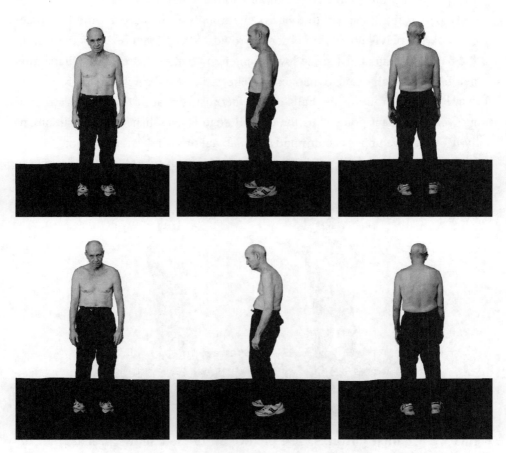

**Figure 21: Showing a normal natural stance (top row) and the combat adjustment (bottom row).**

lightly tighten in and up. (Some schools caution against this, i.e. Cheng Man Ching's Yang style Tai Chi Chuan. I guess they just seal the hui yin cavity, CV-1 between the genitals and the anus.)

The arches are active (use the foot plant you are exploring) and some feeling comes from the ground up the inside of the legs (adductor muscles) to the center of the body and up to the spinal column. This links the actions of the foot and inner leg to the psoas and other inner core muscles.

If you are an external/biomechanical or an internal/energetic practitioner, those centers, mother line, etc. visualizations specific to you would apply here.

Apply your critical edge understanding to the situation at hand.

My personal combat posture has been strongly influenced by the ball practice. I tuck the pelvis up a lot in order to provide a "cup" that receives the weight of the ball. This cup is just at the lower center and makes that center visualization easier both statically and dynamically. The tuck also brings the body weight forward very naturally to the balls of the feet just forward of my preferred bubbling well foot plant point; thus the critical edge is established almost automatically if I focus the upper center/mind on an actual or visualized opponent.

Manipulating the ball with the middle center then makes center integration

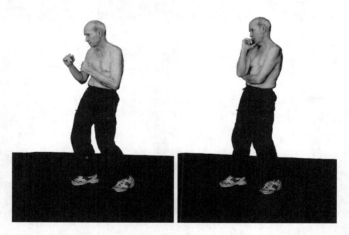

**Figure 22: Combat postures. The picture on the left shows preparation for the start of a fight. The picture on the right shows a proactive posture that can be used in a social gathering when the discussion becomes heated.**

quite easy (relatively) since, as stated elsewhere, the ball is a kind of biomechanical lie detector that can clearly reveal deviations from good body action for correct balance points, proper expansion and contraction, etc.

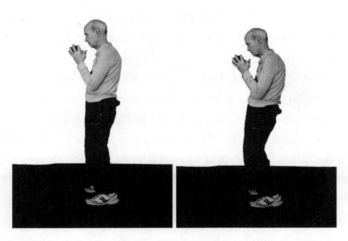

**Figure 23: Pelvis tuck to provide a "cup" for the ball, in natural stance.**

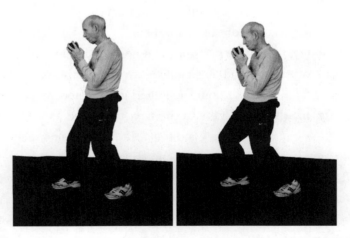

**Figure 24: Pelvis tuck to provide a "cup" for the ball, in front stance.**

# Flow

Pictures in martial arts books frequently show techniques in terms of the beginning and the end of the technique. In reality the problems of balance, posture, timing, etc. occur throughout the whole movement and are best illustrated by a moving picture. Effective structure is a constant and should always be maintained. This is crucial in combat and also important in a form/kata. These are obviously not a series of stop-motion movements, physically or mentally, although that is typically how they are taught and corrected in many styles. In actual application, stances, for example, are not posed and static, they are fluidly passed through.

Maintaining effective structure is more difficult while in the middle of a movement. Movement implies momentum. Controlling ball momentum plus body momentum (which may have differing vectors) helps enhance the ability to control momentum and thus allows for effective mobility. ("Effective mobility" is defined as readily moving on the critical edge with good structure — there will be more on the important concept of the critical edge later in the book.) After training with the ball for a time, one comes to appreciate that the ball never stops and, if the center is moving the ball as you maintain the critical edge, fluidity is much enhanced and dynamic structural integrity becomes easier to maintain.

Critical edge fluidity brings an enhanced mobility in the sense that simply moving the mind brings the body with it. One frequently hears of the body/mind connection. This seems to be one aspect of that.

As stated above, the ball never stops and neither should the mind. The mind is slightly ahead of the ball and never lingers over a past motion. This would be an interruption of the flow. In combat, lingering on a technique just executed, however briefly, interrupts the flow to the next technique and inhibits opponent awareness. This is obviously not a good thing. In fact, keeping the mind ahead of the ball and not just registering its action has a direct combat application. Quoting a famous Yagyu style swordsman, "If your mind follows every changing indication on the part of your opponent that means you are lagging. The thing to do is to force your opponent to follow your changes and, by following his resultant changes, to win." This quote is so good that I use it again below.

With regard to the above quote it is clear that the nuances of ball awareness and the critical issue of opponent awareness are related in that the mind, in both instances, leads. In the maneuver section of the book there are drills with both the ball and an opponent requiring the multi-tasking leading of both.

For another example, and an important one, if you find your breathing interrupted, even slightly, by holding your breath or expelling air more forcefully than necessary when you raise the intensity of your ball movement, try a lighter ball until the fluidity of body, ball, and breath is uninterrupted while maneuvering with intensity. Ideally you can smoothly go all out during a ball exercise with measured and uninterrupted breathing. These mental and physical flow interruptions should be searched out and dealt with before they become incorporated into your technique. It should be emphasized that good flow results from a correct mental structure that moves the physical structure fluidly.

The ball, staff, and empty hand forms (katas) described in this book are training vehicles to develop physical and mental flow and are useful benchmarks to monitor progress.

## Transitions, Transitioning, and Transition Point

Transitions are changes, such as from expansion to contraction, coiling to uncoiling, hard to soft, right side to left side, and defense to offense. Transitioning is the quite nuanced mental and physical process of the changes. The transition point is the specific point at which the change can or actually does occur.

Transitions are an extremely significant consideration for martial arts practitioners. For example, note the emphasis, space, and detail accorded to the subject in *Karate-do Kyohan* (page 211) by Master Gichin Funakoshi of the Shotokan style.[3]

There are times, depending upon the moment, or adjusting to a changing situation, when the defensive hand becomes an offensive hand. This is called "hente" ("changing hands"), and fre-

---

[3] From *Karate-Do Kyohan* by Gichin Funakoshi. Translated by Tsutomu Ohshima, published by Kodansha International Ltd. Copyright © Kodansha International Ltd., 1973. Reproduced by permission. All rights reserved.

quently in actual cases it is more effective than the orthodox use. The effective use of this technique will indicate one's technical level.

The front hand held in defense and the hand held back in offense are variously contrasted as follows:

front (defensive hand), rear (offensive hand)
death hand (shi-te), life hand (katsu-te)
female hand (me-te), male hand (o-te)
yang hand (yo no te), yin hand (in no te)
regular hand (sei no te), irregular hand (ki no te)

It has been said by our elders that "the essence of combat lies in between sei and ki [or the regular and the irregular], and without attaining the ability of changing sei into ki and ki into sei how can one attain victory?" And also, "As yin and yang have no beginning, and movement and non-movement do not appear, who can win but one who knows the Do [way]?" Thus since the essence of karate is found truly between ki and sei or between in (yin) and yo (yang) those who study karate must diligently muse upon these words.

Master Funakoshi's emphasis in the above is on changing and between. One can conclude that transitions or transitioning is a key element in achieving a good level in combat. In fact you could say that the main emphasis of his statement is on the word "between." Be between, for example, offense or defense, ready to react as circumstance dictates. Be able to remain mentally and physically on the transition point "between" while maneuvering against the opponent. Staying on the critical edge would seem to be basically the same concept in terms of balanced orientation to an opponent.

The complete boxer (Western) would be capable of maneuvering seamlessly between offense and defense, able to attack an opening, beat an opponent to a punch, evade and simultaneously punch, counter, or block and counter. This boxer, therefore, would usually be mentally and physically on the transition point, poised, ready, and able to instantly act as circumstance dictates.

If you want to see these abilities demonstrated against dangerous opponents, study the fights of Sugar Ray Robinson and Willie Pep.

NOTE: The Lu Wen Wei exercises in the preliminary exercises below are designed in part to effectively study transitions and transitioning in concert with his multiple centers concept.

## Cardinal Principles

Most "traditional" styles of Asian martial arts have some version of the three cardinal principles: expansion and contraction of the body, hard and soft techniques, and quick and slow movements. For example Shotokan Master Funakoshi cites three cardinal points on page 40 of *Karate-do Kyohan*. Wan Lai Sheng has six energetic principles divided into three pairs: hard and soft, full and empty (distinguishing yin and yang, etc.), vertical and horizontal (slanted above and below; no elaboration on this). Most importantly for this book, Lu Wen Wei's exercises offer excellent practice of the expansion/contraction principle in concert with many other significant concepts.

The forms in this book are observably rich with expansion and contraction. In those parts of Wan Lai Sheng's book that I had translated for me there was no specific information on how the movements in this form could be applied to study the other two principles. I did not want to invent a fixed version of them. I felt that would be too limiting and pass up a chance to work with my understanding. By varying the tempo and intensity of the movements and by using applications noted in other forms, one can create and work with the other two principles while doing these forms.

Practicing with the cardinal principles in mind offers a framework for exploring the forms and combat drills. We can communicate with the old experts by experiencing the application of their concepts to their exercises.

For example, contraction can yield a deadly form of yin energy called "cold" energy. Quoting my brother Curt Adkins regarding cold energy:

> It actually is one of the most easily taught energies once a person has achieved a certain level of relaxation, i.e., no local power in execution of technique. Of course, as in all things in the internal mode, there are levels of execution. The more complex your inter-

nal expression, the more energy. "Cold" energy is most easily developed through sinking and a simple whole-body sink (vertically downward) is translated into approximately horizontal energy — it goes both outward and downward — and when it hits an appropriate target, there is a lot of energy transmitted. Weapon speed is a factor, so a fist as compared to a shoulder can have different targets. This is a matter of skills, though. To paraphrase Yang Zheng Fu: the average practitioner does what he must; the skilled practitioner does what he will.

My Shotokan Karate group strongly emphasizes this same relaxed sinking of the hips in teaching certain nuances of executing effective techniques.

## Breathing

Breathing is a Big Deal. However, with regard to breathing, you will get much, frequently contradictory, information, depending on who you are talking to. Some are not willing to talk about it at all. Most would agree that breathing is a key to connecting body and mind in the execution of technique. The internal stylists will say that breathing is a critical element for chi training. Some of the most important information about breathing are the "do nots" because incorrect breathing can really mess you up.

Actually it all seems to work quite well within the context of the individual style. If you are lucky, you will find a genuinely knowledgeable person who is willing to give you some specific information and exercises/drills instead of cryptic, vague, or ambiguous platitudes.

Abdominal breathing, where inhalation starts by expansion of the abdomen, is the normal method for most martial artists. Another normal practice is exhaling with every technique. I want to explore other possibilities, too, because there are some other effective ways to breathe.

### Reverse Abdominal Breathing

Reverse abdominal breathing, where exhalation is accomplished by expansion of the abdomen, and which I learned about from a genuinely knowledgeable person, was an immediately productive concept. This is a quite comprehensive approach to the mind/breathing process.

Reverse abdominal breathing is a common concept in the internal arts. One application is to settle and manage chi. The Hsing Yi style uses reverse abdominal breathing to store chi in the marrow and to lead chi inward and outward.

Here is information on reverse abdominal breathing from an internal practitioner. (The Mantak Chia book, see bibliography, also has very good reverse breathing information.) From *The Root of Chinese Qigong, 2nd Edition* by Yang Jwing-Ming:[4]

The Reverse Abdominal Breathing method is commonly used by Daoist Qigong practitioners, and so it is often called "Daoist Breathing." Since you are moving your abdomen you are getting the same health benefits that you do with the Normal Abdominal Breathing. However, in Reverse Abdominal Breathing, when you inhale, you draw the abdomen in and hold up your hui yin cavity or anus (Co-1, conception vessel one on the acupuncture charts). When you exhale, gently push out your abdomen and hui yin cavity or anus. There are many reasons for this. The main ones are

1. Greater Efficiency in Leading Qi to the Extremities. Whenever you exhale you are expanding your Guardian Qi. When you inhale, you are conserving your Qi or even absorbing the surrounding Qi into your body. Experience teaches that when you intentionally try to expand your Qi during exhalation, it is easier to expand your abdominal muscles than to relax them. Try blowing up a balloon, and hold one hand on your abdomen. You will find that when you blow out, your abdomen expands rather than withdraws. Or imagine that you are pushing a car. In order to express your power, you have to exhale while you are pushing. If you pay attention to your abdomen while you are doing this you will realize

---

[4] *The Root of Chinese Qigong, 2nd Edition*, Yang Jwing-Ming, YMAA Publication Center, Inc., 1989. pp 129-131. (Reproduced with permission of YMAA Publication Center, Inc.)

that your abdomen is expanding again. If you pull your stomach in when you are doing this, you will find there is less power and that it feels unnatural. Now imagine that you feel cold and want to absorb energy from your surroundings. You will find that your inhalations are longer that your exhalations, and that your abdomen withdraws when you inhale rather than expands. Daoist Qigong practitioners have found that whenever you try to intentionally expand or condense your Qi, you abdomen moves opposite to the way it moves during normal breathing. They realized that reverse breathing is a tool and a strategy that you may use to lead the Qi more efficiently. You can see that the foremost advantage to the Daoist Reverse Abdominal Breathing is its ability to lead Qi to the extremities more naturally and easily than is possible with normal abdominal breathing. Once you have mastered the coordination of Yi, breath, and Qi, you will be able to lead Qi to any part of your body.

2. For Martial Arts. The internal martial arts training of the Daoists is more advanced than that of the Buddhist or any other style. This is simply because the Daoists learned how to lead Qi to any part of the body more efficiently than any of the others. The key to this success is Reverse Abdominal Breathing.

3. For More Effectively Raising the Qi in Marrow/Brain Washing Qigong. In Marrow/Brain Washing Qigong, Reverse Abdominal Breathing is able to raise Qi from legs to the brain more efficiently than the Buddhist methods.

Although there are many advantages to Reverse Abdominal Breathing, there are also several disadvantages or problems which arise during training. Qigong practitioners who use Daoist breathing should be aware of these potential problems, especially during the early period of training. The major problems are

1. Tensing the Chest. In the reverse training, when you inhale, the diaphragm moves down while the abdomen is withdrawing. The drawing in of the abdomen generates pressure upward, which

makes it harder for the diaphragm to move down. This can cause pressure and tension below the solar plexus, which leads to Qi stagnation. This is especially common with people who have just started doing reverse breathing.

This pressure below the solar plexus may cause problems such as diarrhea, or even chest pain. The tension and pressure may cause the heart to beat faster. When this happens, the body becomes positive, the mind is… confused, you become impatient, and your will is unsteady.

This does not advance your Qigong — it makes you sick and hinders your training.

Many Qigong masters will encourage their students to practice Normal Abdominal Breathing until it feels natural and comfortable. Only then will they encourage Reverse Abdominal Breathing. Reverse Abdominal Breathing starts with a small abdominal motion in coordination with the breathing.

During practice you must always pay attention to the Middle Burner [from the solar plexus to the navel], keeping this area relaxed and comfortable. After a few months of practice, you will find that there is a point of compromise which allows reverse breathing to be deep and which also keeps the chest area relaxed. When you reach this stage, you will have grasped the key to Daoist breathing. After you have practiced for a long time, you will realize that your mind does not have to be in conscious control of your breathing. It happens naturally whenever you are practicing Qigong.

The final stage of Reverse Abdominal Breathing is moving your abdominal muscles like a rotating ball. Because the ball is round, your breathing no longer causes any tension in the Middle Burner area. If you train patiently, you will eventually be able to use reverse breathing naturally all the time.

2. Holding the Breath. Because reverse breathing can cause tension and generate pressure in the chest area, people will

sometimes unconsciously hold their breath. It is very important that the Qigong beginner understand that holding the breath while practicing is very harmful. There are some exercises in which you hold your breath, but unless you are doing these specific exercises, you should be careful to keep your breathing smooth and steady.

NOTE: Since the above Daoist material has important implications and valuable applications for martial artists, its study is highly desirable. I do feel that its study should be undertaken only after reasonable martial arts proficiency is attained. There are good reasons to be a bit cautious with breath regulation.

Reverse abdominal breathing came rather easily for me, although there still are problems with consistency when I am focusing on other parts of practice. I found myself going back and forth between the methods depending on the other concepts, which sometimes was a bit distracting. Simply working on reverse abdominal breathing facilitated a breakthrough for me by broadening my views on breathing. If reverse abdominal breathing is too distracting when you practice, I suggest that you make it a separate project from the structure, flow, maneuver, multiple tantien focus of this book.

Another way to solve problems with consistency is to concentrate more on unregulated or non-programmed "natural" abdominal breathing, as described next.

### "Unregulated" breathing

Consider the many styles that insist that execution of a technique must be accompanied by an exhalation. This is easily manageable in the training hall. However, in real combat, possibly against multiple opponents, it is a virtual certainty that you will often need to know how to execute effectively on an inhalation (probably many times).

After working on this for a while I found myself able to do it reasonably well. In fact, expanding into some techniques with an inhalation really seems to work better. There was a smoother flow in some circumstances as well as a more natural expansion/contraction application while making contact at close quarters when sparring.

Many experts speak of smooth, even, "natural" breathing and of just walking around "naturally" without fixed structural considerations during martial arts practice. I have seen some superior practitioners whom I am pretty sure were actually doing this. For me, that was usually very much an either-or, off-and-on situation. However, since becoming more familiar with a broader range of breathing concepts, I feel that I have begun to seriously "taste" these very desirable goals with fair consistency. Some exercises that will help explain the concept further are included in the later sections of this book.

My long-term goal is effective, unregulated reverse abdominal breathing; at some point I will consistently achieve it. The important point though is that whatever martial arts breathing method one ends up effectively using, it must accomplish the goal of connecting body and mind well enough that the mind no longer needs to monitor breathing.

Exploration continues; it's definitely another work in progress.

## Initiators

Early on in practice with the Shaver brothers our focus on one-motion, non-telegraphed techniques led to concentration on the role of the hands, feet, and the withdrawing side (although we weren't calling it that at the time). We had been working on pivots in forms and on evasions while sparring and thinking about the specific use of the withdrawing side in such actions. We were well aware of the relationships of opposite-side hip and shoulder, knee and elbow, etc. but achieving a consistently effective, non-telegraphed, whole-body movement in certain maneuvers was elusive. Then Dave commented on the role of the feet and hands when initiating movements in fencing. Combining the two ideas made a real difference in mobility.

Later when working with the ball I discovered that a one-motion, whole-body movement was more easily achievable if I simultaneously included a hand and foot impulse. It did not have to be a gross movement as long as it included the fingers and toes. Usually just a subtle pulse is sufficient. It was particularly effective when on the critical edge. At present, these are usually automatic initiations for me. If I find myself feeling a bit disconnected, checking the initiator situation frequently relieves the problem. My strong interest in the role of the feet in biomechanics and on foot plant stems from this. I am currently using a modified bubbling well foot plant for most situations; the bubbling well point as the origin point of the spring/shock absorber/engine with the ball of the foot as the main contact/fulcrum and the toes as initiators of foot action and of the lower center.

I feel that the hands initiate Lu Wen Wei's middle center. Intent from the upper center initiates all systems. Ideally these are all virtually simultaneous initializations. Integration of the systems/centers is through the mother line and its extensions.

It was gratifying to subsequently read in William C.C. Chen's three nails article the following, "The fingers [act] to move palms and fists, and body follows." (See http://www.williamcccchen.com/3nails.htm)

## Rebound

This is energy or force from your techniques that comes back to you. It can have either positive or negative results. On the positive side, some of the dynamic offensive or defensive entering techniques rely on taking a bit of rebound to stabilize one's self in maneuvering and to maintain flow.

Negative rebound is the villain. The energy from a deflected or blocked technique coming back to you at unfortunate angles can result in you executing a disruptive technique on yourself. This rebound can interrupt breathing, flow, and balance. The energy from the balance recovery mechanism of a missed technique is another kind of rebound that can result in a self-inflicted disruptive effect. Learn how to recognize when the applied technique has accomplished what it can or cannot do and seamlessly relax into the next technique or a defensive move. This maintains your flow and your opponent connection. I can still hear my early karate instructors say, "Learn to take power off" and my boxing instructor say, "First learn how to hit, then learn how to miss." Rebound understanding is required for effectiveness in both flow and maneuver. Learning how to manage rebound is extremely important.

Some styles have excellent drills for learning rebound management. Most of these are two person drills. There is a one-person practice with a striking bag that has a lot to offer. It is on page 226 of this book.

# Chi

As with internalizing, chi has aspects of structure, flow, and maneuver. Chi is discussed here because if it belongs any one place, flow is the place. Balancing and managing chi energy flow is the linchpin of traditional Chinese medicine and internal martial arts styles. I think that viewing chi in terms of flow makes the application of the concept to structure and maneuver, if only as a visualization, fairly easy and logical.

Chi knowledge is one of the major benchmarks for the internal stylists. When I visited Japan to continue my training in 1961, I attended a gathering with some of the most senior students of Shotokan master Shigeru Egami and asked them what chi was. The group included some very learned academics who were also serious martial arts practitioners. They said that was a huge question and that they thought there were 18 different aspects of chi. I may not have gotten the specifics of the translation right, 18 aspects seems like a lot. At the time this sounded far too complex for me. While briefly studying Tai Chi Chuan in 1959 with Huang Wen Shan, he defined chi simply as intrinsic energy. I still like this definition because it encompasses the extensive variety of chi information without demanding specifics, which inevitably include a mass of contradictions.

Bioelectric energy is another definition that sounds reasonable, simple, and accurate for plants and animals.

Practically speaking, martial artists can forget chi as a general, universal concept and limit their inquiries to human martial chi and qi gong. Within those parameters there is good information with knowledgeable people who can demonstrate and provide exercises and drills that can set you on the path. Although, as with breathing, you may have to sort through a lot of bafflegab before you find the right sources.

Much chi information comes with study of the center. On a beginner level the torso or tantien pumps the chi throughout the body. Advanced skill draws the chi from the tantien. For example, the hand siphons chi from the tantien.

The goal is to generate the chi with the body gradually learning to pinpoint the flow more accurately with less apparent movement. As skills develop, body movement becomes minimal and the mind/intent is used to send chi to the weapon. A minimal amount of movement needed to achieve the maximum result is considered a great goal. All of this while remaining relaxed. Eventually you get to the point where you can issue energy from any position, even a beaten posture.

The above effective beaten posture end point is a good description of successful internalizing for either the internal or external practitioner and indeed should be a very important goal.

Moving chi seems to be a very effective, intuitive visualizing aid for the internalizing process by internal practitioners; external practitioners get there with center and other visualizations, and good biomechanical understanding.

There is an effective introductory exercise for developing the ability to "move chi" in the preliminary exercises section below.

The Mantak Chia book has comprehensive chi management information, which is organized very usefully.

The Hsing Yi book describes chi points, vessels, gates, and channels that are similar beyond coincidence to the mother line with extensions, foot plant points (the bubbling well/kidney 1), and other concepts also used by many external stylists; most are cited in this book.

Quoting from page 4 of the Hsing Yi book[5]:

> In your body there are twelve Chi channels which function like rivers and distribute Chi throughout your body. There are also eight "extraordinary Chi vessels" which function like reservoirs, storing and regulating Chi in your body. One end of each channel is connected to one of the twelve internal organs, while the other end is connected to either a finger or toe. These twelve Chi channels lead Chi to the twelve organs to nourish and to keep them functioning properly. Whenever the Chi level circulating in the channels is abnormal due to stagnation or sickness, one or several organs will not receive the proper amount of Chi nourishment and will tend to malfunction.

---

[5] From *Hsing Yi Chuan, Theory and Applications,* Liang Shou-Yu and Yang Jwing-Ming, published by YMAA Publication Center, Inc. Reproduced with permission of YMAA Publication Center, Inc.

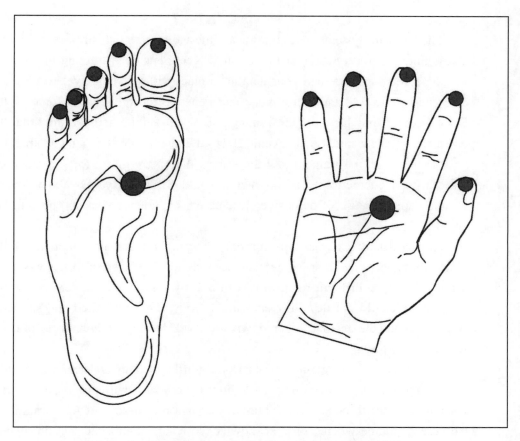

**Figure 25: Location of the chi gates on the hands and feet.**

The eight vessels include four in the body and four in the legs. These vessels store Chi, and are able to regulate Chi flow in the twelve Chi channels. In addition, there are five gates through which the Chi in the body communicates with the Chi in the surrounding environment, and further help regulate the body. The main gate is the head. There are four secondary gates: a Laogong cavity in the center of each palm, and a Yongquan cavity on the bottom of each foot. The tips of the fingers and toes are also considered lesser gates and help with the regulation of Chi.

A way to practice chi flow using these gates is described on page 128.

The Russian Systema martial art is an internal system that stresses energetics study. Intent is a key word for them. Ian O'Keefe has been training in Systema for some years and has had considerable contact with Mikhail Ryabko the head of Systema. He told Ian that anyone can generate the remarkable force of the Systema art if they have proper training and absolute faith and certainty that the objective of their intent will occur. He told Ian that mystifying the arts was wrong; however, the training and the effects they were going for sure sounded like chi-type energetics to me. When Ian told Mikhail Ryabko about Master Egami's apparent use of defensive chi (see chi experiences below), he said "of course."

A great many external-type martial arts practitioners are skeptical of the entire chi concept and many others are accepting but indifferent. It appears to be a fairly long and difficult road. Most of the truly formidable fighters within the internal styles did not develop very quickly. If you are untrained and suddenly worried about the maniac biker down the road, boxing and/or target practice would be the way to go.

I personally am accepting and far from indifferent. This is because I and several of my training partners have had "brief encounters" with chi. Also, my profession as a health consultant continually brings me in contact with traditional Chinese medicine where chi is acknowledged as an established fact and where chi management results in very effective medical treatment. In fact I believe that the practitioners of traditional Chinese medicine have the most comprehensive and accurate knowledge of all regarding chi.

At the very least, the chi idea can be an effective visualizing aid for martial artists.

Gathering information on the subject and working with the information has become an important avenue of my basically external practice. As I said, I have had some chi encounters and soon hope to gain enough competence to justify considering it a reliable part of my combat resources. Next are some thoughts on chi from other practitioners I greatly respect.

## Doctor Akagawa

When I visited Japan in 1961 to continue my karate practice, I was introduced to Dr. Akagawa. He was a medical doctor and an expert practitioner of Iaido, the sword art. Apart from any application of chi in his Iaido practice he also used chi in his medical practice and he offered to demonstrate chi flow to me. He started by pointing the fingertips of his opened hand at the opened palm of his other hand at a distance of about six to eight inches. After a few seconds he was satisfied with his calibration or whatever it was and took my wrist in his target hand, pointed his fingertips at my palm, then moved them slowly back and forth across the width of my palm. I felt a very distinct, cool, focused sensation moving back and forth across my palm. It was about the size of a stream of water coming out of a water faucet. He was not breathing on my hand or moving his "chi" hand fast enough to generate an air current. I had to conclude that it was definitely something tangible and probably was what he said it was.

I have had people demonstrate chi for me by placing their quite warm hands close to my skin. The sensation of considerable heat was definitely there but the question I always had was whether they were really generating chi or demonstrating the well-known ability to control blood flow.

The heat thing raises questions but a cool flow is really much harder to doubt.

## Hayward Nishioka

Hayward Nishioka is an outstanding, long-time Judo practitioner. He is also a black belt of long standing in Shotokan Karate. In 1961 he went to Japan to study Judo and also practiced with Master Egami's Shotokai Karate group. When he returned, I asked him about the practice he experienced with Master Egami's group. Among the experiences he related was one in which he faced another student at close range who had a boken (wooden sword). The other student would hold the boken aloft and then suddenly strike at Hayward's head. Hayward was supposed to dodge the sword. This was anticipation training. After he became proficient at this he was told to turn his back to the sword holder and still dodge the sword. I am sure you will understand that I had some reservations when Hayward said that he had learned to do this. He readily offered to prove it, so there I was standing behind him at a range close enough to bring the sword down on his head with only a very slight sliding step forward. I was willing to smack Hayward but not really hard so I started a bit tentatively. I was not really out of the gate when he whirled out of the way. I ended up trying for maximum stealth and quickness, sneaking up a bit before starting, etc., but as soon as the stroke started, he was gone.

I gave up and demanded to know how he did it. He said that he would feel something hot at the back of the neck and reflexively moved. The feeling was obviously coming just before I moved and probably when I decided and my feeling to attack manifested. I believe that this was an example of defensive chi understanding.

Master Egami is known as a true expert of chi demonstration and obviously can also teach others chi applications as well. In his book *The Heart of Karate-do*, originally published as the *Way of Karate*, on pages 116 and 117 he describes this practice.

### Systema energetics examples

Martin Wheeler has demonstrated energetics application by affecting body parts of persons around four feet away whose backs were turned to him. The knee, elbow, etc. would twitch or otherwise move. The targeted body parts were chosen by a third person. This was witnessed by Ian, Chris, and Dave at a public demonstration. Not all persons were affected, but enough were to be quite convincing. Those who were not affected, someone conceivably standing around "zoning out" or waiting for a heavy tap on the body, would probably not register what is a fairly subtle effect.

- - -

I feel that some "chi" attributes like the above examples are really part of the normal human sensory equipment. They do require good instruction and a lot of work to be practically utilized.

As an example of this, the experiences of a fairly typical group of Californians should be persuasive. A bunch of us were taking part in a segment of the bodyguard training course led by former Green Beret dude Tom Muzila.

Stalking sentries and standing sentry was the exercise. We were taking turns stalking and being stalked and learned that being sharply focused on the sentries soon created uneasiness in them, even when there was a lot of noise from the wind and the birds. They would usually start to seriously look around. We had already learned how to step with minimal noise and with the ebb and flow of the ambient noise. When we defocused our eyes, just keeping the sentry in our peripheral vision, and mentally including the sentry with the surrounding terrain without singling him out, we were increasingly able to complete successful stalks. A few, however, became more difficult to stalk; obviously their awareness was being enhanced in the same way Hayward's was when training with Master Egami's Shotokai group. All of us "got it" to a greater or lesser degree.

Tom has also had good success training SWAT team members and sheriffs deputies to sense whether or not there is someone behind a door and, if so, which side they are on. I am very sure that this inherent sensitivity to the attention energy of others is the same that is so successfully trained in various ways by some martial arts experts.

This also is encouraging as a first step for those who are interested in exploring the broad spectrum of chi applications in the martial arts.

## Empty Arm Punch

There are two interrelated concepts that cross the gamut of structure, flow, and maneuver; these are the empty arm punch and internalizing. I feel they should be discussed before the more performance-based subject of maneuver is considered. This is because the learning curve on ball-related maneuvering is typically not steep until some reasonable familiarity with the ball is attained. Discussing these important concepts before starting to work with the ball ensures that these critical elements for deeper understanding are confronted at the beginning of the process where they belong.

I am using the term "empty arm" in the sense of non-striving, relaxed, and with absence of tension or local power; not as the more commonly considered arm that is not attacking. The "empty arm" is an extension through which the core energy of the feet, legs, hips, torso, and shoulder girdle is transmitted. Effective application of the empty arm punch demonstrates a true understanding of internalizing one's technique. It does not have to be a punch. It can be any combat move applied to the opponent, but the strikes demonstrated by various experts are probably the most graphic and illustrative of the concept.

In his Ball Book Lu Wen Wei provides exercises that are truly excellent in studying and developing this concept. The empty arm punch is extremely effective, can be devastating, and is found as a major goal in a diverse grouping of martial arts styles: Chinese, Japanese, and Russian.

It is a seemingly effortless move that once "tasted" cannot be denied or forgotten. It can be linear or circular and frequently its seeming softness looks innocuous and this is sadly disarming for the recipient's defensive sense, because then the taste test occurs. Here are some examples from several types of practitioners.

**Master Shigeru Egami** was an extremely skillful and dedicated practitioner of Shotokan karate. He is acknowledged as being among the very best of Master Funakoshi's students, a formidable fighter with a lot of practical experience. His studies led him to invite people of many martial arts styles, including boxers, as well as powerful lay persons, to strike his body. He was struck many thousands of times without much, if any, apparent effect. He was beginning to question the whole training process when a junior showed him a seemingly soft punch that was shockingly effective. They worked together on this and the result was a punch that could disable or even kill.

One of the ways Master Egami demonstrated the penetrating effect of this technique was to stack three students in a row. The students had folded karate uniforms on their abdomen. The students behind reached forward and pulled those in front together into a single unit.

Master Egami stood before the group in a front stance with his fist just touching the folded uniform. He then executed his technique, just suddenly reaching forward, which folded all three and was felt as a shocking abdominal blow by the last student. He was eventually able to transmit shock through more than ten people to a single point in the body stack. The persons all had thin pads on their abdomen to ensure a continuous line of contact through the group for the punch.

We first heard about this back in 1963 and Mr. Tsutomu Ohshima, my instructor, tried it out on two students. One of these was my own student, Bob Lopez, who was the rear victim and who felt a sharp punch at a single point on his abdomen. He felt ok at the time but woke up that night in considerable

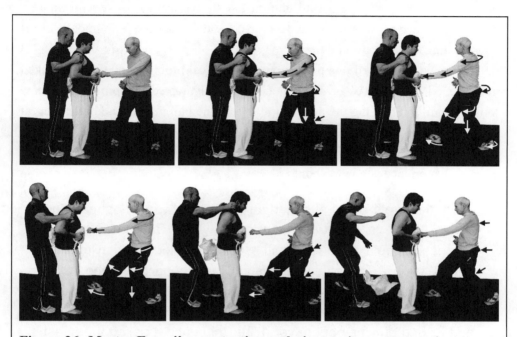

**Figure 26: Master Egami's penetrating technique using a contracting, cross-loading application of the empty arm principle. See page 33 for the application using the expansion principle.**

**In picture one a neutral position is shown. In picture two weight transfers to the rear leg as the lower center drops and the middle center rotates around the mother line with impetus toward the target. In picture three the lower center continues to sink strongly as the right leg steps powerfully through the target. The middle center simultaneously rotating around the mother line cross-loads with the lower center through the target. The right leg and left arm are leading the integrated centers here. Body contraction is quite apparent at this point. In pictures four and five force has been transmitted to the target as the puncher continues the "step" through the target. Focus remains on the target. In picture six the step is completed.**

physical distress.

This became a regular part of our practice. Mr. Ohshima tried up to three people quite successfully, the rest of us just one person. Sometimes we could achieve a truly penetrating punch, sometimes not. Besides the standard punch we tried palm strikes, backhand, and bottom fist strikes from very short distances. The key to success was to be quite relaxed and to just make a smooth effort coordinating mind, body, and breath.

I personally stopped this practice when physical problems due to my broken neck forced me to focus on resolving the steadily worsening problems. I now look forward to applying the new insights from the ball practice and other recent information to a renewed study of the concept.

The Tai Chi Chuan style has a similar concept as described by Curt Adkins after his experience at a workshop:

> In the late 1970s I attended an East Coast workshop featuring a very high-level guest instructor of a style of Tai Chi Chuan that emphasizes relaxation and softness, a so-called "yin" style. After one session a few of us were standing around doing the usual post-session "talk boxing." The subject of punching came up and I mentioned that I had experienced being hit with gongfu, karate, and boxing punches but never a Tai Chi punch. I asked the guest instructor if he would mind providing an example of a Tai Chi punch and offered my right shoulder as a target.
>
> The host instructor was embarrassed by the request but the guest instructor merely chuckled and stepped close to me. He lifted his right arm, bent about 90 degrees with a standing fist about shoulder height but the elbow quite low. The fist was only about 2-3 inches away from my shoulder. There was no sensation of a punch-like movement, just a slight shift of his body. The hit felt solid but shallow on the shoulder, though going to my center. There wasn't any push or follow through.
>
> Later, a couple of people asked me what it felt like and I said that the guest instructor obviously was merely humoring me without wanting to do real damage. Then I asked them what the punch

looked like. One said that he just seemed to raise and lower his arm without really doing much else. The other said that he watched the shoulder for movement but only saw the body turning slightly with no apparent movement in his arm or shoulder, except to move toward me.

The next day I noticed four blue-green bruises on my shoulder, corresponding to the four knuckles of a fist. These then developed into one rather large blue-green bruise, bigger than a fist. Over a period of several days the blood in this area eventually drained down into the lower arm. As I recall there really wasn't much swelling in the shoulder, though, just a lot of subcutaneous bleeding from tissue damage.

Many years later I again experienced this instructor's energy, this time a shoulder strike to the chest. It hit my centerline just above the sternum and was like a sledgehammer blow going straight through to my feet. I was stunned and unable to move for several seconds, though I didn't go down. Again, there was minimal outward movement and no real sense of a "local" hit though it affected my whole body. There was no push or follow-through, and there seemed to be minimal contact. This time there was no bruising.

**Systema** (a Russian martial art) Masters Mikhail Ryabko and Vladimir Vasiliev both discuss and display how power comes from proper breathing, movement, and posture, not overt strength and speed. Many professional and high-level martial artists have commented on the shocking power of their strikes that were seemingly "empty" of any tension.

Chris and Dave Shaver received strikes from Mikhail, Vladimir, and Martin Wheeler and were extremely impressed with the shock effects.

Chris did an exhibition bout with Mike Weaver at the time Weaver was heavyweight boxing champion and has sparred quite a lot with ranked professional fighters so he well understands the relative power of punches. The Systema punches were casually and apparently rather lightly rendered but the effect was profound.

Dave experienced some "soft" palm strikes from Martin that were shocking and left his whole body feeling bruised.

The above empty arm examples lead one to the question of how effective their own techniques really are. An honest answer for a great many would probably be "not very" or "I am not sure."

Another consideration along these lines is, assuming that your technique is effective, applying it on an opponent that does not want you to and who is presently trying to apply his technique on you, will no doubt render your efforts problematical. Drills, exercises, etc. that address these considerations will be included in the discussion of maneuver.

## Internalizing

These empty arm techniques are a prime example of internalizing ability and understanding. Those who have effective empty arm abilities have internalized their technique to a very high level. They demonstrate the difference between effective technique and lethal technique. I feel that an accomplished internalizing ability includes a deep understanding of the interrelated rebound management, withdrawing side, and core energy transference concepts coupled with proper breathing. I had been aware of the concepts but until I made quite a bit of progress with the ball work, I had not begun to realistically implement them.

Rebound management was discussed on page 54. To briefly summarize, it involves the management of force/energy returning or coming to you from contact with an opponent in such a way that your flow, critical edge, opponent orientation, and force application is maintained or enhanced.

The withdrawing side, simply stated, is separated by the mother line from the advancing side in technique application. Both sides may be advancing, but one, often the attacking side in combat applications, advances more. This frequently results in more emphasis and thus thought and feeling placed on the advancing side. This can lead to incomplete application of the entire biomechanical arsenal available for combat applications. For example, the multi-vector rotating ball center visualization is a layered sphere with a center point located on the mother line. When executing techniques, the sphere rotates around the center point. The center point can be considered the mother point. Obviously each side of a vector in any given rotation around the mother point is of equal significance and must be accorded equal consideration. Noting the benefit of added attention to the withdrawing side in executing a series of uppercut-hook combinations on equipment held by a training partner will confirm this.

For a very common example of successful internalizing with correct core energy transfer and withdrawing side use consider the walking illustration on page 72. The whole body is advancing forward, but the complex biomechanics involved result in opposite hip and shoulder, knee and elbow, and foot and hand alternately and momentarily moving forward just a bit more and faster than its opposite on the other side of the mother line. These opposite numbers are the withdrawing side. Both the inner core and outer core muscles of the torso are transferring their energy efficiently to accomplish this and the other body parts and mechanisms (foot action, cranial/cervical junction, etc.) are well integrated with the core to transport the body. This all occurs without conscious biomechanical thought, breathing is natural, and the mind/intent is on the destination and the "room." As far as walking is concerned this is successful internalizing.

Unsuccessful internalizing while walking is very common and can be observed on a daily basis on any street or in any mall. A few minutes observation reveals many people who walk holding their upper bodies still and progress by kicking their feet forward. There is no fluid balancing of opposite hip and shoulder; basically the whole body advances forward as a solid unit. The inner and outer cores are minimally involved in the basic human activity of locomotion. Since walking the streets and malls is typically not a critical situation, unsuccessful internalizing there is a non-issue; obviously combat is a different situation entirely.

The far more complex maneuvers of combat require a much more detailed understanding of the internalizing biomechanics involved for successful application of internalizing to techniques involving coiling/uncoiling while contracting and/or expanding, along with proper martial arts breathing. A maximum understanding yields a maximum survival potential.

The various exercises of the maneuver section are designed to progressively introduce the elements for good understanding in a sequence that evolved based on feedback from training partners.

Combining various visualizations with ball work and practical exercises such as heavy bag work has helped my understanding considerably. Among several useful studies of internalizing, I have been visualizing the mother line and the centers as the "core," core energy transfer as energy out, and negative rebound as dark energy in. The withdrawing side is involved in managing/utilizing both.

The result of this study has been a much increased appreciation of internalizing. I have come to feel that internalizing is one of those "gateway" concepts that lead to the truly significant questions. Based on one's martial arts background, the gates will no doubt vary a bit and thus the questions as well, but I strongly feel that the internalizing concept is of major significance for serious martial arts practitioners. Please keep this point in mind when working on the exercises in the maneuver section.

There is more on internalizing in the Advanced Drills section.

# *Maneuver*

The third of the three important concepts introduced in this chapter is maneuver. As stated above, maneuver is strategically oriented; opponents are involved. The opponents can be real or visualized (shadow boxing, forms), or equipment such as striking mitts, bags, and fight shields can be used in a strategic format.

The static combat structure is relatively easy to visualize and utilize. The dynamic combat structure (maneuvering) is not always that easy to consistently maintain, especially if things are not going well. Effective maneuver requires understanding of centering, the critical edge, flow, "room" and opponent awareness, offensive/defensive transitioning, the three cardinal principles, breathing, and rebound management.

Successfully incorporating these into your martial art techniques with a true opponent connection takes a lot of work, but is fairly doable considering the large number of drills and exercises available to us.

The mental, strategic, and tactical elements of maneuver are another side of the game. This is an area that ideally combines strategy, tactics, mentality, and mindset, including understanding that is derived from real-life experience. Here the thoughts of someone who did this for a living are particularly apt. For example, on the critical subject of opponent connection: "the readiness to regard any change on the opponents' part as coming from you is of primary importance. If your mind follows every changing indication on the part of your opponent, that means you are lagging. The thing to do is to force your opponent to follow your changes and, by following his resultant changes, to win." This is from the Yagyu family *Book on Swordsmanship*, quoting Yagyu Munenori. The quote applies very broadly; I used it in another context above. Other examples are in the books listed in the combat mentality and training section of the bibliography. The books provide an excellent combination of theoretical and practical information from proven fighters who devoted their lives to the subject.

If you maneuver well and your strategy and tactics are sound, a final consideration is the actual effectiveness of your blocks and attacks on your opponent. Core energy transference, withdrawing side, rebound management, disruptive techniques, and internalizing techniques such as the empty arm are at the heart of this problem. The advanced exercises, based on ball and other related practices, are intended to teach these concepts.

Many of the topics required for effective maneuvering have been discussed already. In this section I want to add information about awareness, disruptive techniques, and centering.

## Awareness

I once had the opportunity to ask Master Ohtsuka, the founder of Wado-ryu karate, how much attention to focus on the opponent and how much on everything else. He said that was an important question. His answer was 80% for the opponent, 20% for everything else. I assumed that 20% meant fighting surface, other people relatively near, etc., in other words "the room." I would assume that these ratios would vary with your familiarity with the combat environment and the opponents.

Free-for-all sparing with the staff against several opponents soon teaches you the critical importance of seeing, feeling, and hearing the "room." In a melee the more functional your peripheral vision is, the greater your survivability. Multiple-opponent sparring is also a very good test of your ability to remain mentally "centered." When you practice with real opponents in a melee, these problems become obvious. As experience is gained, proficiency comes.

Individual practice of forms or techniques is another matter. One should learn to execute movements without being internally focused. Be able to visualize opponents and also see the "room." Fight your way through the form or technique.

Of course monitoring your structure, timing, balance, etc. for self-correction is vital. So a large part of your practice will have this internal focus. One should, however, also be able to do an effective individual practice with a mentality and external mindset as close to reality as possible. Work for the ability to effectively perform an individual practice (forms, shadow boxing, etc.) against visualized opponents as fast and as intensely as you fight or spar with real ones. Your success with this can and should be checked by executing the same techniques against training partners with and without equipment. The feedback you get here will improve your self-practice ability quite a bit.

Self-awareness is an important consideration with various nuances on several levels. The old Chinese and Japanese masters have left us a lot of relevant thought on the subject that deserves serious consideration. In real combat being too aware of one's "self," even a little bit, can be another dangerous inhibition or even a fatal distraction. One's comfort level with damaging others is a very basic consideration. The subject of centering below deals with more of these considerations.

## Disruptive Techniques

These are destabilizing techniques that attack the opponents' structure, balance, or orientation instead of vital points. For example, a lot of the two-handed/augmented-hand techniques in the martial arts forms are disruptive, as are many of the rising blocks that attack Lu Wen Wei's middle center (for example). You can certainly not forget sweeping techniques. While not necessarily decisive, disruptive techniques can be very influential in the outcome of combat.

The ball practice is very good for working on two-handed techniques, and the ball momentum and balance management work yields an enhanced anti-disruption defensive sense.

Many of the drills in the sparring and mobility drills section below are good for working on disruptive techniques. With a good partner you can trade roles as attacker/defender and partner/disruptor to study the offensive and defensive aspects of disruption. Obviously rebound management has its role here as well. Practical applications of disruption techniques are effectively studied in sparring, the staff sparring being particularly well suited for this.

## Centering

Centering is a commonly used term in many styles with various nuances in meaning. By centering I mean simply the following:

Centering, the verb, means strategic application of the centers and/or the mother line while executing techniques in combat. For example, maintaining effective orientation of your mother line to your opponent while maneuvering in combat, being mentally centered, or the application of what my brother calls the "cross-loading harmony" of shoulder with hip, knee with elbow, and hand with foot (or wrist with ankle). They cross load at the center. This cross loading is the balanced way we walk.

Cross-loaded centering is important for learning the empty arm punch and for withdrawing side and other internalizing techniques.

Grapplers seem to intuitively gain a good understanding of the centering principle. I believe this is due to the close range nature of the grappling arts where destabilizing offensive and defensive technique is taught and applied almost from day one.

A true principle will apply to all the martial arts. For example, I recently had the opportunity to train with Bobby Taboada, Grand Master of the Balintawak Escrima Cuentada style of Philippine martial arts. His stepping and striking drills, in particular, drew on the same centering ability/knowledge as the ball, and

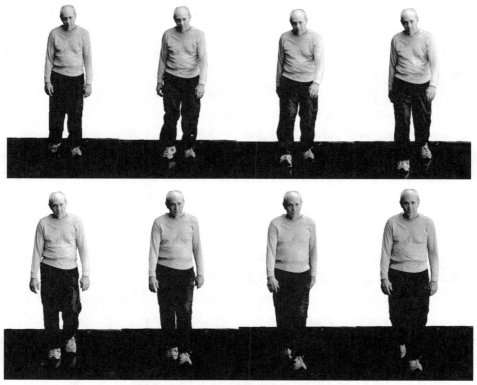

**Figure 27: Cross-loaded walking.**

were a quite superior method of inculcating those principles into one's technique. In fact, after this six-hours-plus seminar I found that the same centering muscles I was most aware of with the ball exercises had been so heavily worked that they were nearly depleted. My mother line awareness was enhanced and it also seemed that the centering had become more unconscious and automatic.

This is the ideal. As with any visualizing aid, once integrated and automatic, the mind will not need to be focused on it and will be free to deal with other things. Like opponents.

Being centered mentally is another aspect of equally critical importance in combat. Mental and physical tension slows reaction time, execution time, and impairs judgment.

If you are mentally centered, you can be focused without being fixed, be intense without being tense. This is not terribly difficult to accomplish while sparring with friends in the training hall or opponents in a sporting match. Real combat, where death or disability is a very possible result of failure, is another matter entirely. The knights-errant of China and the samurai of Japan paid a lot of attention to this problem. I particularly enjoy their efforts to settle their mind and to deal with ego. They improved their mentality to improve their martial arts and they improved their martial arts to improve their mentality. Perfect symmetry.

Practice active stillness since if you are shouting, you cannot hear. Listening energy, number 39 of the *T'ai Chi Boxing Chronicle* in the appendix, refers to this point and succinctly states its practical application.

Even if you do not contemplate such serious encounters, this really is a path to technical improvement.

There are a lot of excellent books that deal with this aspect. The bibliography lists several. They contain concepts and considerations such as seizing the chance ahead of time, attachment, and lingering, which are important to understand in improving combat ability. This material really deserves careful consideration.

Sparring with multiple opponents is very good training for, and a practical test of, your level in this.

The maneuvering drills in the Sparring and Mobility chapter introduce the ball and weapons into maneuver practice.

# 3. Preliminary Exercises

## *Equipment*

You will need iron balls of various weights. Shot puts of a large variety of weights are available from athletic supply firms. The weights to use depend on your size and strength. Personally I use a six-pound iron ball so I can go all out moving around with no danger of losing control. This controllability is important if you are trying out new ideas or some of the more gymnastic maneuvers. My eight-pound ball is right on the edge of controllability. The ten-pound is not reliably controllable during maximum effort. My twelve-pound ball is currently the heaviest I feel comfortable training with.

Each weight has its place and will teach you different things. For example the heavier weights are very good for training and ingraining a fluid whole-body technique. The lighter weights can allow arm or upper body over-emphasis to pass unnoticed. I am of average size and strength, so choose your ball size accordingly. Do not use the smooth, polished shots as they are too slippery. A small person could start with a four-pound ball. The

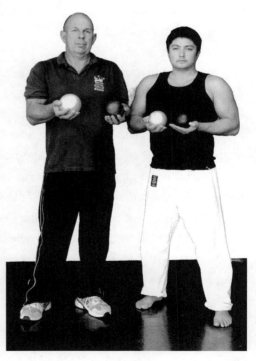

**Figure 28: Different sizes of iron balls.**

websites at the back of the book list shot put sources.

Lu Wen Wei mentions many wood and metal balls of varying weights. The weights of the balls cited in Wan Lai Sheng's book were approximately 16 and 20 pounds. My brother sent me a DVD clip of a man named Chen Qing Zhou who uses a 14-kilogram (30.8-pound) ball, which he manipulates against his body (mainly the tantien area) and which he throws surprisingly high into the air and catches in the course of executing a form. Call me a sissy but I feel this is too much unless you are a 300-pound lineman for the Pittsburgh Steelers.

With regard to the weight of the balls, I have gone through some changes in my practice. I started with a light ball, trying to soften my body and keep the weight from tensing my body, either generally or locally, as I increased the vigor of the movements. As I gained proficiency, I increased the weight and was able to maintain the body softness even with quite intense activity. This was actually a very good plyometric workout and my physical condition improved quite a bit. My maneuverability improved in sparring and all other practice. Eventually, however, I discovered that my body was really not as completely relaxed, fluid, and springy as I wanted.

At the higher weights I could not completely relax mentally and I just could not totally stop "over-managing" the ball. Going to lighter weights let me develop my sensitivity to movement subtleties by comparing the same movements all the way up to the highest intensity with and without a light ball. Currently this is my main emphasis and I am feeling an improved resilience in maneuvering and effectiveness in application of techniques.

I still use the heavier weight balls to review the whole process and to work with certain movement areas that I have identified as personal problems. This is the point. It is a process that individuals can personalize for their own needs.

In addition to technical enhancement, the ball is excellent for pure physical conditioning. It works the body the same way the currently popular Pilates and "core" training systems do while providing a superior cardiovascular benefit.

## *Exercises with the Ball*

### Holding the Ball

Holding the ball correctly is important. The hands form a flexible, sensory cage that is almost exactly the same size as the ball. The upper palms and the fingers hold the ball in a rather liquid, sensitive grip as shown in Figure 29. Do not press or squeeze the ball. There is more about holding the ball in the exercises below.

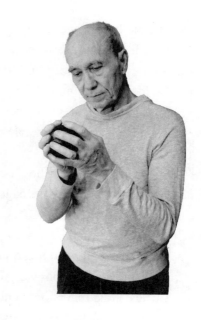

### Movements with a Ball

Once you have a basic familiarity with the exercises below, Start to integrate the following points into your practice.

There are quite a few points to consider, many will no doubt be familiar and already integrated into your technique. Others may be unfamiliar, defined differently by your own style, or be considered irrelevant. They have all been cited at some point above or are expanded upon at a few places below.

Obviously thinking about many concepts at once is ridiculous, but awareness of the more critical concepts to explore is important for progress. A personalized, prioritized list can be very helpful, especially for new material or different approaches. Here are

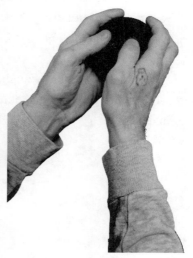

**Figure 29: Holding the ball.**

some of the significant considerations I think you should keep track of as you practice the exercises. Add or subtract from the list as required.

- Mother line awareness (with extensions) is a constant.

- The mother line generally aligns with a visualized opponent.
- Withdrawing side awareness is a constant.
- Mother line/withdrawing side relationship, a very important study.
- No local power, no local power, no local power.
- Springy, resilient, whole-body force application is a goal from the outset.
- The three cardinal principles, especially contraction and expansion.

If you are unclear on how I am using some of these terms, you may check the definitions of them on these pages:

Flow, page 43.

Breathing, general, page 48.

Unregulated general breathing, page 52.

Daoist reverse abdominal breathing, page 48.

Critical edge/transition point, pages 15 and 45.

Rotating ball centers visualizations, pages 26 and 39.

Foot plant and bubbling well, pages 26 and 28.

Internalizing, pages 66 and 230.

All the non-opponent visualizations and considerations, such as those listed here, once integrated and automatic, can lapse into the background and eventually fade.

## Figure-8 Movement

Start with a light ball, about six pounds. Hold the ball in front of you at about throat level with the elbows just clearing the chest.

The hands do not press or squeeze the ball. Use a tactile grip, feeling that the hands are a flexible, sensory cage that is almost exactly the same size as the ball. The upper palms and the fingers hold the ball in a rather liquid, sensitive grip as shown.

As you can see from the illustration, this is quite analogous to the bubbling well location in the foot plant. The fingers initiate, the "ball" of the palm is a main contact/fulcrum, and the P-8 (laogong chi gate) point energizes.

The eyes follow the ball. At first look at the ball to check your grip and hand motion, later defocus your eyes somewhat to bring your peripheral vision into play.

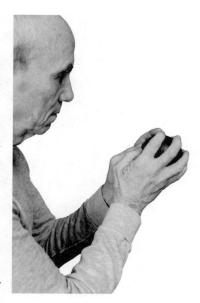

**Figure 30: Starting position of the ball for the Figure-8 Movement.**

### Tracing the weight/energy vectors

Soften the body. Assume a combat posture. Let the weight of the ball pass down the shoulder girdle into the lower abdomen/center. Straighten out the lower back a bit by tilting the pelvis up slightly to "catch" the ball. THE center, as described in the section on structure, is holding the ball. A visualization that has been helpful for some training partners is that the pelvis is a cup holding the ball; the center being the cup's contact point with the ball. Losing the tilt of the pelvis empties the cup. Note that the

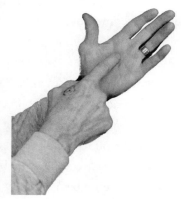

**Figure 31: The location of the pericardium P-8 energy point, which is used to energize movement with the ball.**

pelvis tilt naturally shifts the body weight forward onto the balls of the feet. Support for the body comes up from the ground through your feet to the lower abdomen. The feet should have the same tactile feel as the hands. The arches of the feet are active.

Move the ball from hand to hand in the figure-8 pattern as shown in Figure 33.

The pace is quite slow to begin with in order to clearly note the weight shift of the ball at the feet and the effect of the weight transfers on your visualization of the center.

The fingertips should be active in controlling the ball. This is important. Try to feel that the fingertips are a trigger that connects to the mind to initiate upper body movement. The elbows and wrists are the main drivers for the ball with the elbows making relatively smaller motions. As the size of the figure-8 pattern increases, the elbows are relatively more significant.

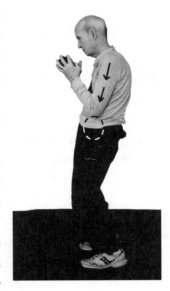

**Figure 32: Adjusted posture for holding the ball with ball visualization.**

Feel the adjustments your upper and lower body make to accommodate the weight shifts as the ball changes hands and directions. Note also that as your hands and elbows manipulate the ball, your feet make subtle adjustments in their contact with the ground. Take notice of the actions of the toes in these adjustments. The more vigorously you move the ball, the more obvious the adjustments become, traveling up through the ankles, knees, and hips to THE center and generating feedback up and down the mother line. This process lets you discover the relationship of the hands and feet with the centers. Trace the most effective paths between them to and through the centers. Be sure to maintain the relaxed, springy softness in your body. Tenseness will obscure the pathways.

**Importance of the feet**

At this point I wish to focus on the role of the feet. Softness of the body is not total relaxation. It is the absence of unnecessary tension. There is a springy resiliency that is required for effective execution of technique in combat. This is particularly true for the feet. The feet, like the hands, are designed for and are capable of a very large variety of biomechanical actions.

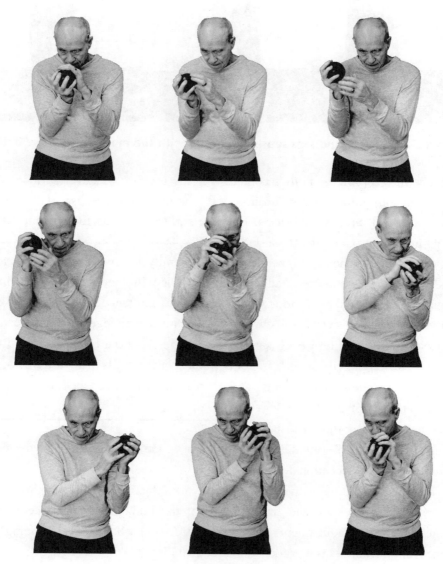

**Figure 33: Performing the Figure-8 exercise.**

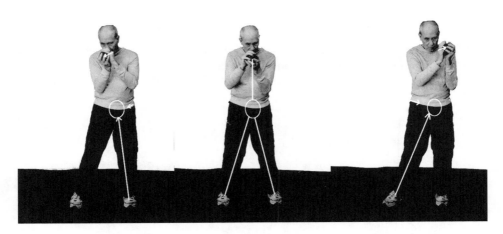

**Figure 34: The feet and legs sense alignment with the movement of the ball.**

Since the feet are the body's contact with the ground, whatever surface you are fighting on, either shod or unshod, there is an appropriate use of the toes, balls of the feet, arches, and heels. Possible surfaces include the training hall, carpet, uneven ground, rough surfaces (e.g., unfinished cement), slippery surfaces, etc. (As an example, to adjust to slippery surfaces soften the foot somewhat and use an even, full-surface contact for extra traction.) Each surface requires a different adjustment in foot biomechanics. These adjustments will work together with the lower legs and ankles to provide optimum response to

> Generally the most useful basic foot plant is with the weight about on the balls of the feet at the bubbling well, but this can change when the surface changes. Try the basic drills and the subsequent drills with different foot plants, shod and unshod, on a variety of surfaces.

any situation. The differing surfaces provide a variety of challenges to the feet and thus a broader educational format.

The ball practice helps the feet learn to work effectively wherever they find themselves. The feet are the first adjustment the body needs to make when changes occur. The adjustments of the feet affect the whole body. Training in differing circumstances is a prudent and practical idea.

The above process is used to determine the paths for loading and moving the ball with and through the center(s) in a martial arts sense.

Next, try initiating body movement up the paths from the ground contact through the centers to the hands. Reproduce the previous adjustment actions of the feet in generating body movement that flows up to the hands. The hands are then initiated by finger pulses that move the ball. Try using the idea of mother line extensions in the legs and arms at this point if you haven't already and if you wish to experiment. Move the hands and elbows as before to control the ball. This is the most common application of force to an opponent in martial arts techniques.

When this becomes familiar, concentrate on feeling that the hands, centers, and feet are acting simultaneously as a unit along the lines of force to move the ball. No local strength should dominate. For example, a change of ball direction does not come mainly from the hands and arms. The springy resiliency moving the ball originates in the centers and is diffused throughout the body. The more effectively you do this, the lighter the ball will seem.

Your focus during this should now be to the front and about where an opponent would be. At some point you should begin to visualize an opponent.

Visualize the opponent moving just a bit from side to side in front of you. Maintain your mother line on the opponent's mother line. Be sure to note the changes in body connectivity and adjust to maintain a resilient unity of hands, centers, and feet for ball movement.

Use a heavier ball and repeat.

Repeat the above exercises without the ball. Try to sense the feet, ankles, lower legs, hands, etc. working in the same way as with the ball.

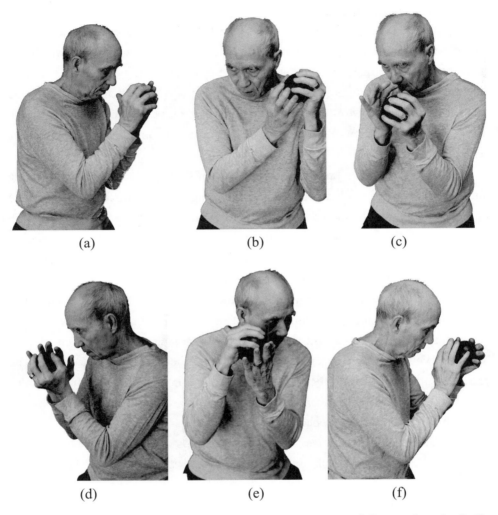

Figure 35: Starting to visualize following an opponent while moving the ball. (a) start, (b) see opponent to the side, (c) follow opponent, (d) continue following, (e) react to a move to the other side, (f) follow.

## Side to Side

Return to the lighter ball. Begin to visualize that the opponent is occasionally moving a bit more from side to side in front of you. Turn to follow while maintaining a steady forceful flow of the ball.

Visualize that the opponent's side-to-side movements are getting larger. As you follow his movement to the side take a small step with him and then back with him as he reverses direction. Note the adjustments the feet make to receive the body shift and then integrate with the centers and hands in order to make a seamless whole-body reversal of direction. Also note the helpful role of the knees as part of THE center in this process.

The lower abdomen, which has received the energy of the ball, has to continually adjust the body in order to maintain the centering on the opponent. The intersection of the adjustment forces is the key physical activity center of the body. Balancing body momentum with differing force vectors of the ball in order to orient your center on the opponent in front of you will become automatic with time. It is important to keep the body soft and especially important not to tense those muscles in the neck and shoulders that raise the shoulder girdle. Undue local tension inhibits the center-oriented resiliency required for core energy transfer and whole-body movement.

Repeat without the ball.

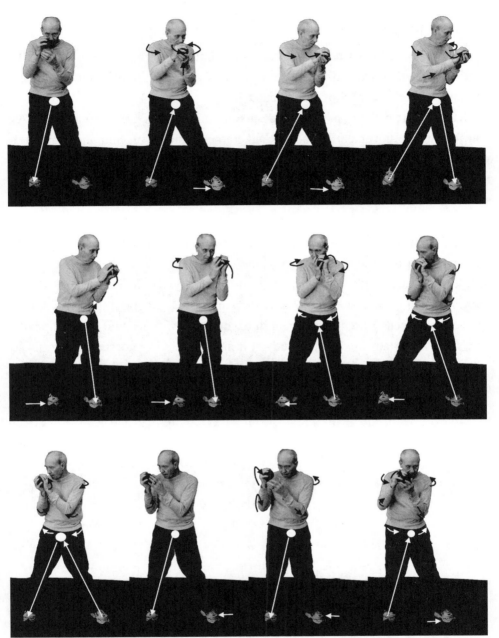

**Figure 36: Following an opponent from side to side with the ball.**

## Rolling

Hold the ball cupped in both hands. Roll the ball in your cupped hands as shown. It is a bit like steering a car but in three dimensions.

Pay special attention to the fingertips. Do not use your forearms as primary movers. Roll more with the fingers and wrists, and use the wrist-forearm connection as secondary movers. Rolling is not as forceful as the larger figure-8 patterns above. The effects are more subtle. It will require more sensitivity to note effects of the forces generated by the ball and relate them to the body's force vectors and center activity.

Repeat the process as in the figure-8 practice — ground contact, opponent visualization, etc. The same considerations as in the figure-8 apply to this exercise.

Repeat without the ball. Pay special attention to detecting the sensations of the tactile feet and hands, which will be more subtle without the ball.

Center awareness and whole-body resiliency is less obvious as well. Being on the critical edge here will help in sensing these and other such important points.

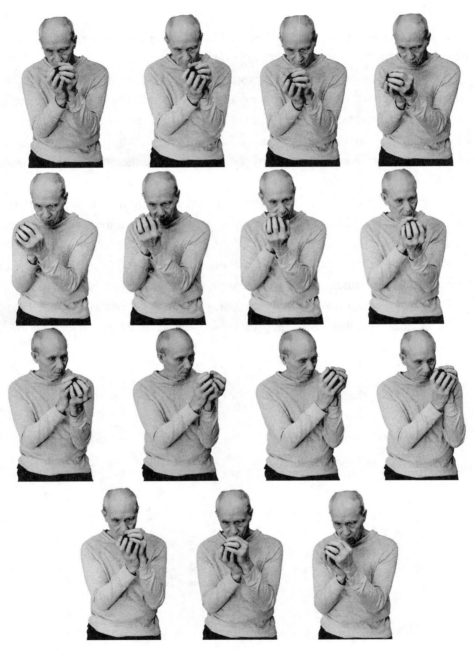

**Figure 37: Rolling the ball.**

## Maneuvering

After learning the basic force/energy centers and the transmission paths required for using the ball, one can apply them to further study of the martial arts actions of maneuver. Turning, pivoting, dropping, rising, coiling, uncoiling, expansion, and contraction are important combat maneuvers. These maneuvers are in all of the forms and exercises to be introduced below.

Maneuvering is really the same as stepping except that it involves complicated changes of direction. It does however require more concentration to execute an integrated "whole-body" maneuver. Moving the body segmentally is slower and less effective. It is also much easier for the opponent to "read" your maneuvers. Ideally the body is integrated in its movement and moves in its entirety all at once in an instant response to necessity. This is achievable if you have a balanced structure on the critical edge to begin with. Using the ball can really improve your understanding of the process. Ideally your fighting movements will eventually come to be "walking" around in this natural manner while executing effective techniques. You will be using your body in the way it is designed to be used.

## Expanding and Contracting

Your body is constantly expanding and contracting in daily use, sitting down and standing up, for example. Combat contraction and expansion equivalents of those would be (for one example) center dropping power and center rising power. The physical structure can also be powerfully contracted/concentrated and expanded/diffused to a certain degree for good effect in the execution of many techniques. Effective contraction and expansion demands a good fluid structure and ready mobility throughout the contractions, expansions, coiling in, uncoiling out, and many, many other maneuvers typically used in combat. Structural adjustment nuances contribute to effective maneuvering. For example, softening the chest and expanding the back is a common structural adjustment for effective expansion and contraction (and for effective technique application in general).

The most accomplished martial artists I have ever seen have shown mastery of this principle. Whether it is a short, precisely penetrating contraction that collapses you or a large, dynamic expansion that sends an opponent flying, to see it or to feel it is to believe it. The Systema practitioners and Master Egami's examples cited above command belief.

Ed Parker's Long Beach, California, tournament in 1964, which introduced Bruce Lee to a large number of us, is another good example of this. He was already impressive up to the point that he demonstrated his one-inch punch, but when Bruce expanded explosively against the chest of the guy who then flew back into the chair placed well behind him (which then slid back a couple of feet), the cake was thoroughly iced.

## Breathing

Breathing would probably be the most fundamental example of expansion and contraction. Breathing is a Big Deal in the martial arts and touches on most aspects of practice. There seem to be a fair number of differing views on the subject. Within each genre, or even each style, you can be given a lot of information, much of which may outwardly appear contradictory, but which usually has its own validity in terms of the genre or style.

Since there is general agreement that correct breathing is important, if not critical, to connect body and mind, it would follow that effective expansion and contraction requires close attention to the subject of breathing. If the breathing is interrupted in any of several ways, there is a problem.

Several generalizations can be made, such as: abdominal breathing is desirable and reverse abdominal breathing is preferable; do not hold the breath or strain to breathe, etc. Smooth, even breathing is emphasized by many and the point is often made that mental calmness facilitates correct, well-regulated breathing and vice versa.

These elements must be integrated with maneuver and with the "fight" the maneuver represents. The forms and many of the exercises below contain a lot of expansion and contraction in their maneuvers and are a good practice for this integration.

# *Lu Wen Wei Exercises*

The following three exercises will develop ball familiarity, work on Lu Wen Wei's multiple centers, and explain concepts about breathing that are vital for progressing with the exercises from the Ball Book that follow. Having these three concepts fairly well integrated is required for quickly learning the depth of understanding available from Lu Wen Wei's exercises.

## Body Shifting Exercises

These exercises introduce mostly in-place body shifting that mainly focuses on the flowing use of the feet/centers/hands while exploring the action of the foot/ankle/calf/knee power train; this is the engine/suspension system alluded to on page 27.

This is also a good place to outline and illustrate basic usage of foot plant action that can be incorporated into the maneuver drills below.

### Holding the Ball

Stand with the weight on the rear (right) leg with the (light) ball cupped in both hands just at shoulder level as shown in Figure 29. Straighten out the curve of the lower back by tilting the pelvis forward and up. The weight of the ball settles to the softened body's lower center. The "cupped" pelvis visualization works well here. Ball weight there should be sensed occasionally throughout the exercise. What you have here is an actual ball held in the middle center, which is activated by the visualized middle center and a visualized ball in the cup of the lower center. This simple exercise sequence provides good insight into the study of multiple centers integration and internalizing. The weight of the body is mainly on the balls of the feet and is on the critical edge.

Do not maneuver the ball at first. Just hold it in the basic combat position while studying the details of foot, ankle, calf, knee, and hip action when shifting the body back and forth.

Shift the body repetitively and seamlessly forward and backward as shown. You may be responding to an opponent constantly edging back then in a bit. Maintain the critical edge as you do this; the pace is smooth and rather slow. Do

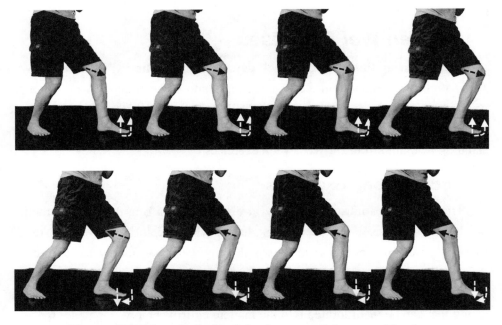

**Figure 38: Using the ball of the foot as a fulcrum, side view.**

not linger at any one point. This is a very small motion, continuously flowing just a bit front and back. Concentrate on the lower legs and feet in order to isolate and study their role in body shifting.

The shifts are accomplished as follows (see Figure 38):

The right foot extends down and simultaneously the left foot flexes up.

With the weight on the balls of the feet, flexing the left foot up with the tibialis anterior muscle will drop the left knee and enable an easy forward impulse of the left hip. Right foot extension is initiated by pressing the toes down with the tibialis posterior and calf muscles, although toe pressing and foot extension are virtually indistinguishable.

A simultaneous forward right hip thrust (hamstrings, calf, quads mainly) shifts the body forward strongly with control and balance throughout the shift.

The weight has now passed onto the front leg. Instant reversal of direction is accomplished by the left leg's toes initiating foot extension down. As stated above, this is a small back and forth flowing series of movements by a fluid body to isolate proper foot action and get a good sense of it.

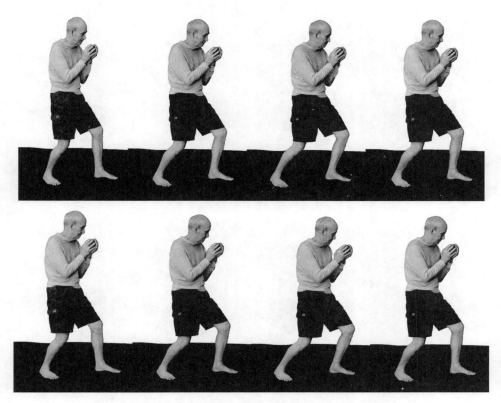

**Figure 39: Shifting the body while holding the ball.**

The weight is maintained on the balls of the feet. When the weight shifts forward the front leg arch lengthens (relaxes) as the left foot flexes up; the rear leg arch contracts (shortens) as the right foot extends down. When shifting forward the weight does not move onto the toes; when shifting back the weight does not pass back onto the heel. This is a good way to really get a feel for the power train/suspension systems cited above.

If you have trouble sensing the foot and lower leg action, try a heavier ball.

**Add Ball Extension**

Next extend the ball forward as the body shifts forward. If you are properly on the critical edge, just a slight forward shift of ball weight will enable an instant whole-body shift. The action here is initiated by simultaneous finger and

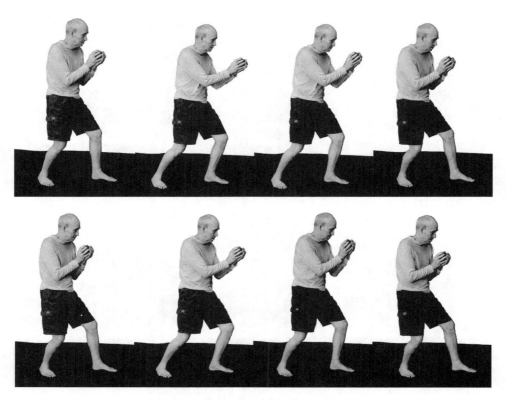

**Figure 40: Sifting in with ball extension.**

toe impulses. The hands use a very slight rolling action cited above and the feet, legs, knees, and hips use the biomechanics studied immediately above.

As the body moves forward, the ball moves forward and down a bit extending out to the front, the body turning somewhat to face front and the weight shifts briefly to the front leg as the ball circles up and around to come back and down with the weight simultaneously shifting back.

### Add Stepping

Move flowingly back and forth several times, then, when you are at the point where you are ready to shift forward, make a counterclockwise arc rolling the ball to bring it to the left side as shown. Seamlessly take a step forward together with the arc and flow into the drill on the other side. Note that there is a middle center action here that needs to be coordinated with the lower center for a whole-body single motion. Stepping forward with the left leg requires a clockwise arcing action.

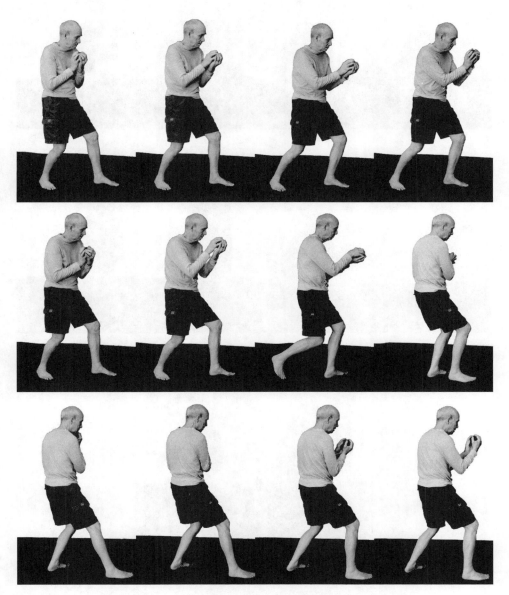

**Figure 41: Stepping forward with the ball, side view.**

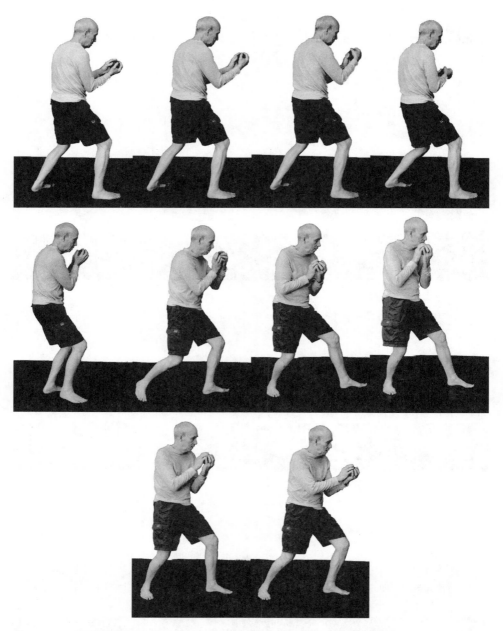

**Figure 42: Stepping backward with the ball, side view.**

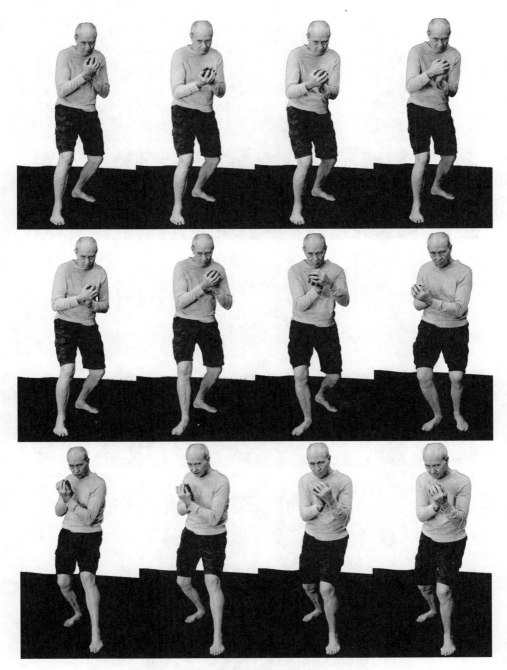

**Figure 43: Stepping forward with the ball, left leg front view. Note the clockwise arc.**

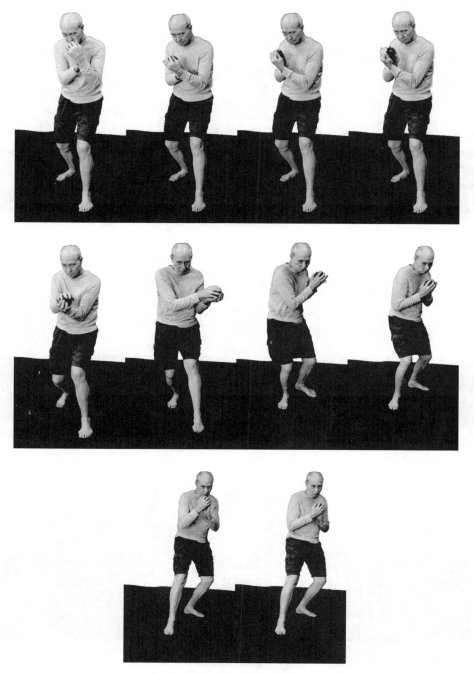

**Figure 44: Stepping backward with the ball, front view.**

NOTE: The withdrawing side is a major element of the shift, engaging the lower and middle centers around the mother line and controlling the weight transfer appropriately with regard to critical edge maintenance.

Add in occasionally stepping back and to the sides at various angles and seamlessly resuming the body shifting. In stepping frontally with a long step, weight passes through the heels of the stepping legs to the balls of the feet. When stepping back, the weight should move onto only the balls of the rear foot and resume the shifting.

The body is seamlessly moving front, back, and around in response to intent, thus all three centers are active in this simple drill. At first the eyes should be focused on the ball and the mind monitoring the biomechanics. When you feel familiar with the biomechanics, begin to visualize an opponent shifting, stepping, and generally maneuvering skillfully around. Respond to the opponent within the framework of the movements above. This is a good exercise to return to for experimenting with basic critical edge familiarization.

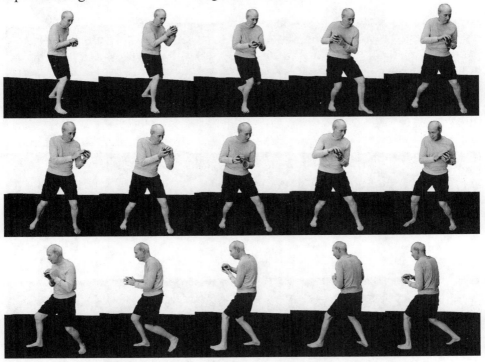

**Figure 45: Stepping in all directions with intent.**

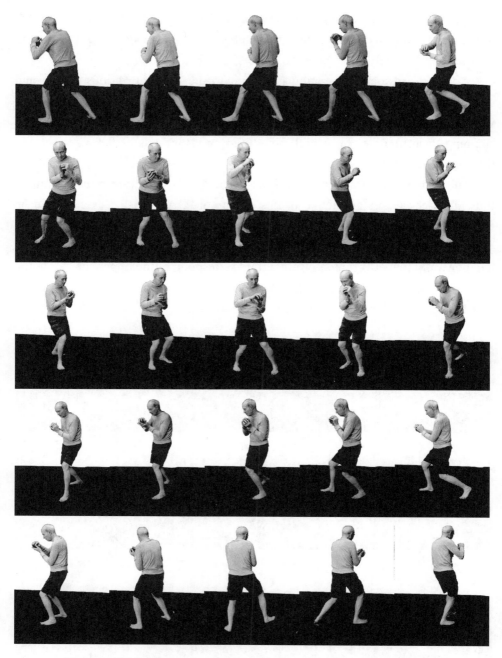

**Figure 46: Stepping in all directions with intent (continued).**

# Center Exploration

### Lower Center

Step forcefully forward while strongly swinging the ball from side to side perpendicular to the body's forward direction as shown. The pattern is right ball movement with right stepping leg; left ball movement with left stepping leg, seamlessly repeating. Rotate the visualized lower center ball in opposition to the iron ball vector.

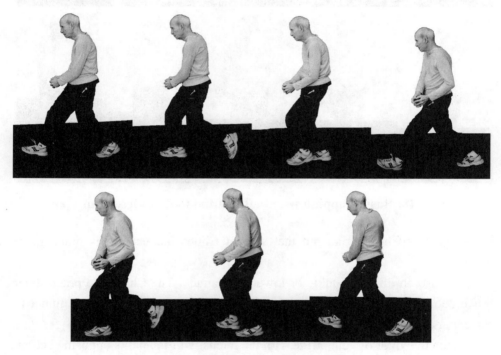

**Figure 47: Basic stepping with ball shifting to the sides, side view.**

When this is familiar, take increasingly longer steps until you are reaching well out with your feet to rapidly stride very forcefully along. The stepping leg action at this point changes to an ankle or foot striking kick with a pronounced heel strike to the ground at the conclusion of the strike. This modification to the basic stepping version was made after viewing a very similar drill from the Ancient Chuo Jiao group on YouTube. (Search YouTube.com for Ancient Chuo Jiao. You should find four videos labeled 1 of 4 to 4 of 4.) Normal stepping has a

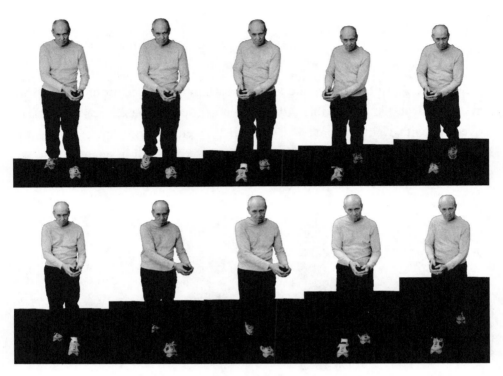

**Figure 48: Basic stepping with ball shifting to the sides, front view.**

non-emphasized heel strike but the Ancient Chuo Jiao version is much more instructive.

It is also an effective ankle or lower shin attack. The Chuo Jiao practitioner broke about 10 tiles stacked against a post. This technique is a nice adjunct to sweeping as a move that attacks a target that tends to be closest to you.

Match the vigor of your stride with the intensity of the ball's opposing action. Match the destabilizing ball action with lower center vectoring. To help maximize the force of your stepping, a forceful, reaching extension of the stepping leg, with a lower-level kick adds a lot.

Also note that the powerful inner core iliopsoas muscle contributes a lot to the cross loading balancing of this exercise. The more forcefully the ball moves perpendicularly, the more forcefully the iliopsoas works leg extension for proper balance.

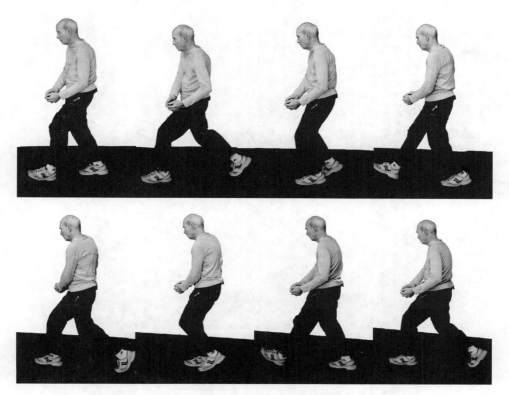

**Figure 49: Forceful stepping with strong cross-vector ball motion.**

Note the role of the leg's powerful adductor muscles to help maintain linear foot tracking.

### Middle Center

Using the above exercise, the middle center can be studied by repeating the exercise and visualizing the middle center mainly or solely while working the ball from the combat position as shown.

Coordinate stepping leg reaching with ball action; this can be cross vector or ball punching. When it feels right, try basic punches with the same timing.

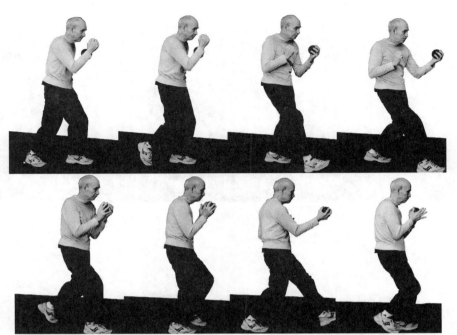

**Figure 50: Middle center practice, stepping with ball punching.**

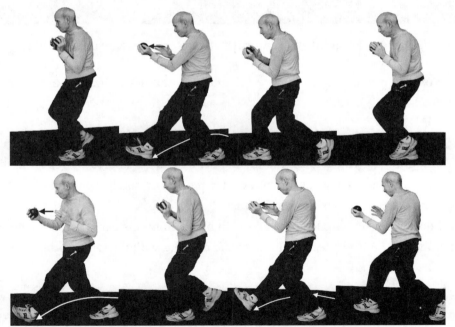

**Figure 51: Middle center practice, heel kick with ball punching.**

**Two handed bag striking with Escrima stick**

With an Escrima stick strike the bag as shown with one hand holding the stick. Note the effectiveness of your strikes.

Next hold the stick with the other hand placed on the wrist of the stick hand as indicated in Figure 53. Strike the bag in the same pattern as before with power emphasis on the withdrawing side. The heavy arrows indicate the withdrawing side; light arrows show the augmenting/uniting/targeting side. Note how the palms basically face each other as in the ball handling. Most note a considerable power increase with the hands united. Integrate the middle center action with the toes, fingers, and lower center all working the stick.

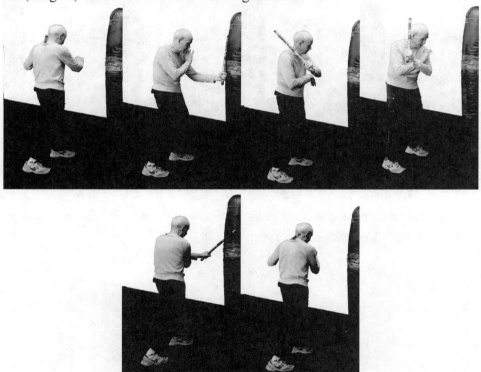

**Figure 52: Striking the bag with an Escrima stick using one hand.**

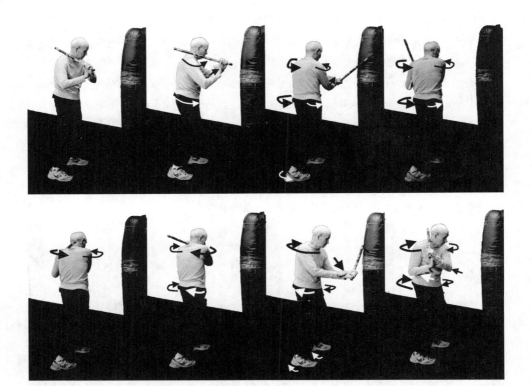

**Figure 53: Striking the bag with an Escrima stick using two hands.**

There is an expanded version of this exercise in the withdrawing side discussion part of the advanced exercises on page 225.

**Stepping with double punch, with and without ball**

When Shotokan Master Egami visited our group in 1973 he executed a two-handed punch from a natural stance that started so smoothly that he was well into the technique before we realized he had started. He said that we should learn to move like that. Legs, body, and hands were one; everything started and finished together — seamless whole-body movement from perfect balanced stillness to perfect balanced stillness. This simple technique struck me strongly at the time and remained a constant in my training.

This exercise and the double hand attack with kick (below), both practiced on the critical edge, are designed as one way to study Master Egami's movement.

The centers, feet, and hands finish the attack simultaneously inside the visualized opponent. Weight and momentum transfer to the front together with the hands entry into the opponent. This means that feet, hips, and hands are all still in forceful forward motion when the hands contact the opponent. Recovery of the hands to the guard position and settling of weight to the front foot re-establishes the critical edge.

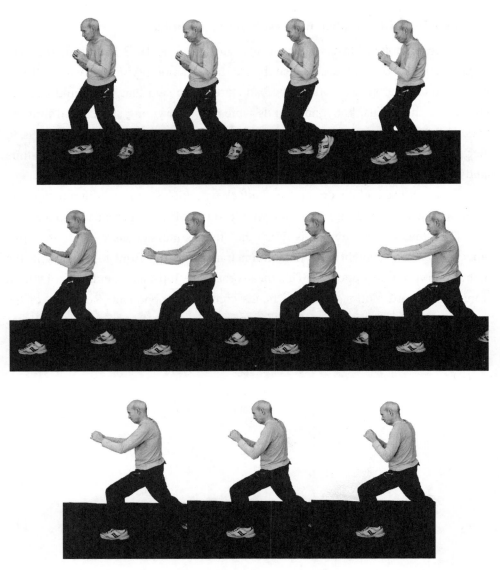

**Figure 54: Executing a double punch with empty hands.**

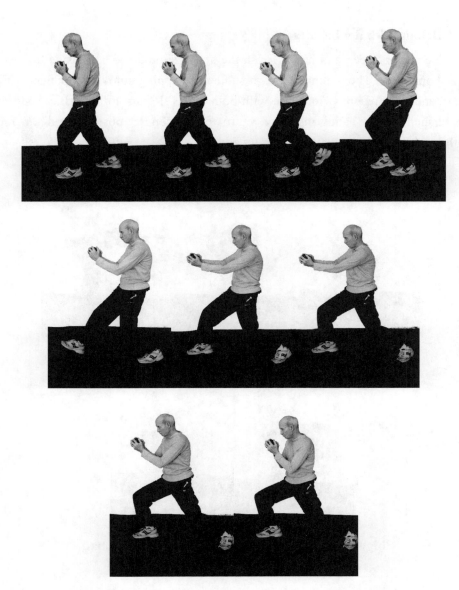

**Figure 55: Executing a double punch with an iron ball.**

### Kicking with double attack

The centers, feet, and hands finish the attack simultaneously inside the visualized opponent. The feeling is that of suddenly stepping onto the opponent while simultaneously reaching into him with both hands. Return to the critical edge is established as the hands instantly return to the combat position and the foot withdraws a bit on the way to touching down.

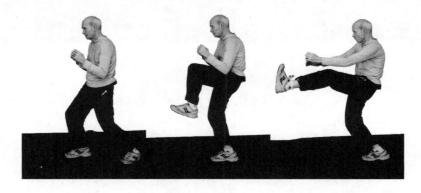

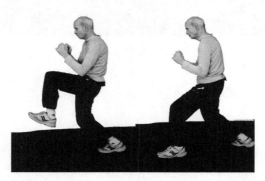

**Figure 56: Kick and double punch without a ball.**

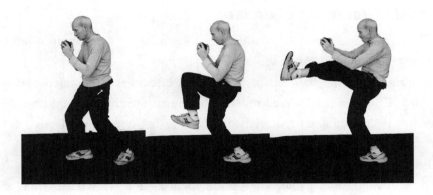

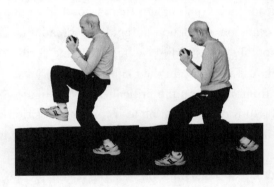

**Figure 57: Kick and double punch with a ball.**

## Basic Breathing Exercises

This is a logical place to consider breathing from the standpoint of breathing as a constant flow united with the constant ball flow.

Working with the ball led to a focus on effective unregulated abdominal breathing. Effective unregulated reverse abdominal breathing would probably be better but is certainly not required for effective ball work or effective combat technique.

I have found that most people get the inhaling execution easily if it is introduced with hip-rising, expansion-type techniques and with basic front kicks. There is a triple front kick combination that is good for a continuously flowing feeling while working on inhalation/unregulated breathing. Perform the kicks while inhaling smoothly and steadily, switch back and forth between inhale and exhale as you work, use inhaling for the majority of the kicks.

From a basic front stance on the critical edge (in Figure 58), execute a rear leg front kick and return the kicking leg to its original position while returning to the critical edge. Then execute a front leg front kick and return the leg to its original position while returning to the critical edge. Finally execute a stepping front kick with the rear leg, finishing on the critical edge. Your have now reversed the initial stance and can repeat the sequence on the other side.

The kicks should be executed without any disturbing effect on the middle center, such as preliminary "wind-up" motions. When the triple kick pattern is familiar, add ball attacks as shown in Figure 59. This adds the middle center to the exercise to check for center integration along with the breath management. Keep the ball constantly moving, synchronizing it with the kicking. Keep the breathing constant, inhaling on the kicks for the majority of the work. Keep your mind on the flow of the ball, staying just ahead of it; move it into the opponent and back to the recovery hand while synchronizing with the centers and the feet. Soon you will become a bit winded and it will become rather easy to disconnect from a managed breathing pattern and just focus on the ball and the opponent without regard to breath timing. The breathing will also begin to come from the lower abdominals, especially if you visualize a pelvic "cup" holding the ball.

After this is familiar, try unregulated breathing with the body shifting and center exploration exercises above. The Escrima exercises are very good once you are starting to really get it. They work the middle center a lot and will also uncover unfortunate tendencies for local power and neck tension in the upper center. Correct breathing really helps to smooth away these types of problems.

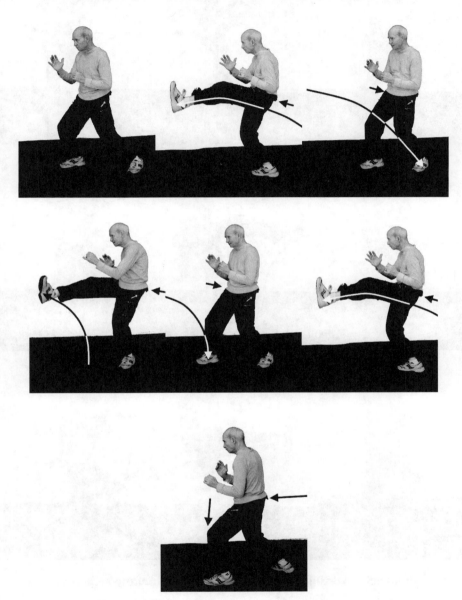

**Figure 58: The basic kicking sequence.**

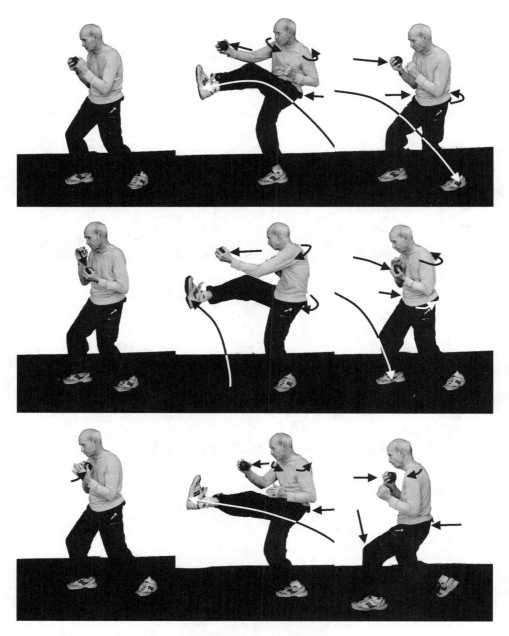

**Figure 59: Adding ball movements to the kicking sequence.**

## Exercises from the Lu Wen Wei Ball Book

Here are three exercises from the Ball Book that are pretty basic and are a good beginning for studying Lu Wen Wei's thinking on the ball. I selected these because of their simplicity and because they have a variety of ball movement directions to manage. They have one of Lu Wen Wei's zan exercises and two of his fan exercises. Seasoned internal practitioners would no doubt get more out of his basic information than us external types. As excellent as his material is, there is not a lot of biomechanical guidance in the manner of more modern books. This is not necessarily a bad approach. You can have some very good insights on the byroads.

I did find some unrelated but productive information while wandering and eventually discovered that the multiple centers concept forced an in depth study that pretty well covered the biomechanical ground of Lu Wen Wei's exercises. The theoretical information and preliminary exercise material above is intended as a shortcut past some of the more unproductive roads and dead ends I pursued over the years.

Once the exercise movement patterns are familiar and a good flow is established, begin working with Lu Wen Wei's multiple center concept. I found that this added substantially to the excellent energizing effect I had noted from working the patterns. This multiple centers concept is unusual, challenging, and potentially extremely rewarding. My training partners and I have benefited considerably from everything we have applied it to so far.

For internal practitioners particularly, but probably for many others eventually, Appendix 1 includes a translation of a part that could be of interest. At the risk of complicating this very basic introduction I will include these definitions of zan and fan right here.

> What are zan and fan? Zan is active; fan is quiescent. What are yin and yang? Zan is yang; fan is yin. Zan starts from the inward and then goes outward and up. Fan comes from the outward and then goes inward and down. In all moves the hands and face are toward each other. When the palm is toward the face, this is yang; when the back of the hand is toward the face, this is yin.

Here is a part of Appendix 1 that pertains to all of us.

In all moves the hands and face are toward each other. The body has three dantian [tantien], upper, middle, and lower. The arm has three joints, wrist, elbow, and shoulder. The hands move in all possible manners scribing large circles of 360 degrees; small circles also have 360 degrees. The large circles are slow, the small circles are fast. Some are shaped; others are formless. In all movements the arms are not straightened and most commonly are bent 90 degrees. This makes the circles lively.

The pace of the exercises will obviously be very slow at first to ensure that the face, the ball hand, and the empty hand are properly oriented and that the ball hand transfers occur at the correct places in the movement sequence.

NOTE: these ball transfers are changes in the exercises from zan to fan and vice versa. These are critical changes and should be energetic, seamlessly flowing, whole-body, and smooth. They obviously have a mental as well as physical component and breathing is a key element. These are the transitions referred to in the quotation from Master Funakoshi on page 45, and they are a true expression of expansion/contraction and other important related principles.

The forms (katas) below contain many technique sequences where these transitions occur and are very good for studying them in concert with the other concepts.

If you are thinking internal and working on the zan-fan, yin-yang material right from the beginning, the pace should be even a bit slower. There is a lot to consider with this approach.

Once you are familiar with a movement and you can make a smooth, even flow automatically with natural, even breathing, you can speed up somewhat for a very energizing effect.

Try increasing the pace. Continue to gradually force the pace as long as you can continue to execute the exercise without breath interruption, local power sneaking in, or loss of the correct face, hands, and ball orientation.

There is no special virtue in being able to go really hard and fast. All speeds should be worked to uncover problems and discover nuances, but all should be explored equally. The various speeds of execution are valuable for differing insights. Ease of working the three centers, foot action, withdrawing side, core energy transference, zan and fan transitions, etc. would determine your choice of pace for the majority of your practice time. Ball weight also influences the pace that is possible or desirable.

Each one of these exercises seems to lend itself to a slightly different pace that seems really "right." Obviously this is a personal observation, but so far it holds true. It would appear that these well-designed exercises are each speaking to the crux of their individual design.

## Ball Posture 1

**Circling above the Knees; this is a zan exercise, it starts inward and goes outward and up, then becomes fan and goes inward and down.**

Take the Opening Posture of high horse or natural stance with the ball in the right hand, step out 45 degrees with the left leg and shift the weight to a forward bow stance while extending the left arm and looking forward over the extended leg. The left arm is bent about 120 degrees palm forward, fingers upward at 45 degrees, and with the little finger at about nose height. The

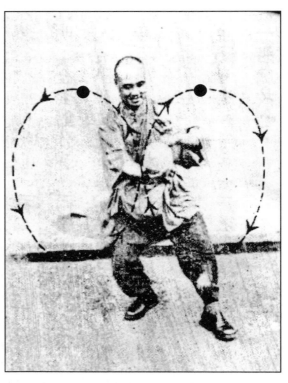

Figure 60: Ball posture 1, Circling above the Knees from Lu Wen Wei, showing the transfer points at the dots. The exercise may also be performed with the arrow direction reversed (ball comes from the outside and down). This variation gives insight into the Lu Wen Wei freestyle.

right hand holds the ball at chest height slightly left of the torso centerline. The left hand is above and left of the ball. The energy is found in the left leg.

Twist to the left and raise the ball toward the left hand. Then transfer the ball to the left hand. This initiates the figure eight path shown in the photograph. At the point of transfer, the thumb of the hand receiving the ball is at about ear height.

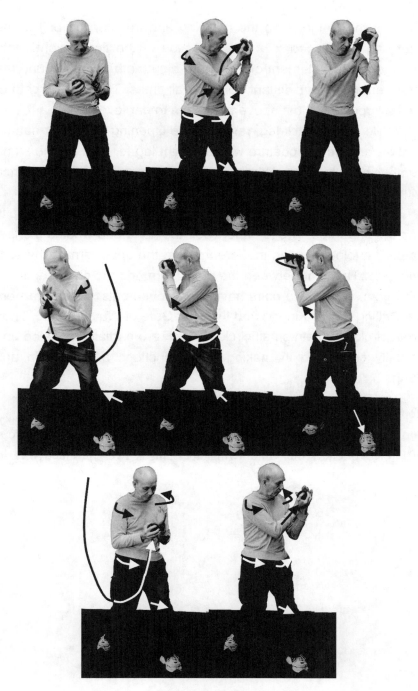

**Figure 61: Circling above the knees.**

Shift the weight onto the right leg and transfer the ball to the right hand at the apex of the right side of the figure-eight. Note that the vertical element of the figure-eight path wraps around the torso remaining equidistant from it at all times. The circular path of the ball goes from just above the knees to ear level.

While on the back leg, return to the Opening Stance or natural posture and do the posture with the right leg forward for the same number of repetitions. When finished return to the natural stance with the ball in the left hand in front of the right chest.

Explanation: The arms have three gates between the armpits and the fingertips. The joint between the hand and wrist is the first gate. The joint between the forearm and the upper arm is the second gate. The joint between the upper arm and the shoulder is the third gate. These two pairs have four movements, which are from the Drilling Fist of Xing Yi and the First Gate of Wu Ji Boxing. Their great circles contain small circles, which are partially revealed and partially concealed in making the distinctions between Yin and Yang.

Repeat without the ball (phantom ball).

Perform the exercise with the ball in the other hand (visualized phantom ball as well) to feel or check the withdrawing side. This is a very productive variation.

## Ball Posture 13

**Pouncing Tiger; this is a fan exercise, it comes from outward and goes inward and down, then changes to zan and goes outward and up.**

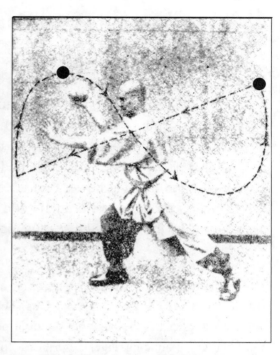

Take a high opening stance with the ball in the left hand at waist height and the right hand opposite the ball palm down. Sink the weight into the left leg, turn the hips to the left, and extend the right foot out at a 45-degree angle. Make a left back stance holding the ball as described. Shift the weight forward into the right leg and sink the ball forward and down at about a 30-degree angle. The right hand is slightly lower. The torso is angled forward forming a straight line with the back leg.

**Figure 62: Ball Posture 13, Pouncing Tiger from Lu Wen Wei, showing the transfer points at the dots.**

See the photo [Figure 62]. The ball is near the top of the forward circle. This posture is called Pouncing Tiger or in literal translation, Tiger Catches Prey.

The ball scribes a semi-circle forward, up, and then back with the body following along and twisting to the left. At the apex of the front circle the ball transfers to the right hand. The body shifts back and sinks into the back leg to make the circle with the ball in the right hand. Shift back while rising and twisting to the left in an arc and transferring the ball to the left hand. Repeat the posture several times.

While in a forward posture with the ball in the left hand, shift all weight into the right leg and step the left leg forward and to the left. Turn the body to the left, transfer the ball to the left hand and repeat the posture on the left side.

Explanation: Throughout the posture the hand holding the ball is slightly higher. The palm of the empty hand is generally facing downward. The tiger's rush is like a mighty wind, therefore in changing directions or turning the body and transferring the ball to the left hand there is power and energy like whirling wind. When the ball is carried by the dragon hand the ball is the jewel; when it is carried by the tiger hand it is the food prey caught by the pouncing tiger.

Translator's notes: The stance starts in a back bow and moves to a front bow stance as shown in Figure 64. (Note that the beginning neutral posture is not shown.) Pouncing Tiger describes a forward leaning bow stance posture with both arms extended. See Figure 63. Dragons are said to guard or pursue a jewel. The jewel is often interpreted as chi.

Repeat without the ball (phantom ball).

Perform the exercise with the ball in the other hand (phantom ball as well) to feel or check the withdrawing side. Again, this is a very productive variation.

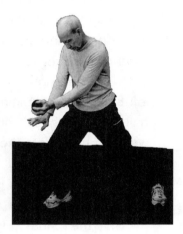

**Figure 63: Showing where the tiger has captured the prey.**

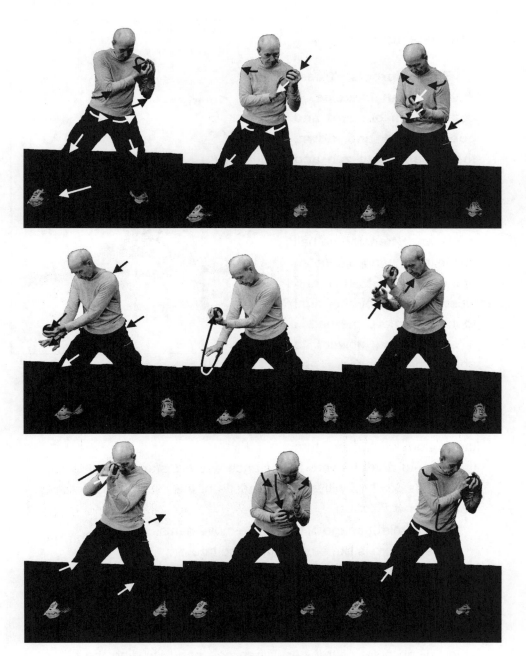

**Figure 64: Performing the pouncing tiger exercise.**

## Ball Posture 14

**Bear Uproots Trees; this is a fan exercise, it comes from outward and goes inward and down, then changes to zan and goes outward and up.**

From the Pouncing Tiger posture with the right leg forward, transfer the ball to the right hand. Make an arc downward to just outside the toes of the right foot. Then move the ball in a straight line upward to above the forehead. Then again downward to the front of the toes of the right foot. Repeat this movement. At the bottom of the arc, turn

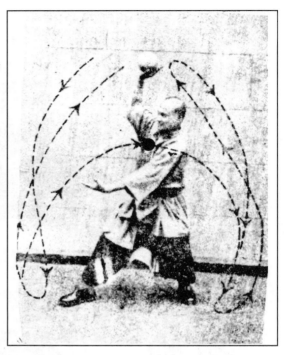

Figure 65: Ball Posture 14, Bear Uproots Tree from Lu Wen Wei, showing the transfer point at the dot.

the body to a left forward bow stance and transfer the ball to the left hand side. This will be the opposite of the initial stance of the posture.

Do the mirror image of the above movements.

This posture is like a bear uprooting trees.

Explanation: In this posture, the stance has the right leg bent and the left leg extended backward [a rather longer stance as shown in the photo] so as to bend down. After the movements are executed with skill the ball may be thrown from one hand to the other at the point of transfer. When one hand is rising the other hand is near the chest or stomach.

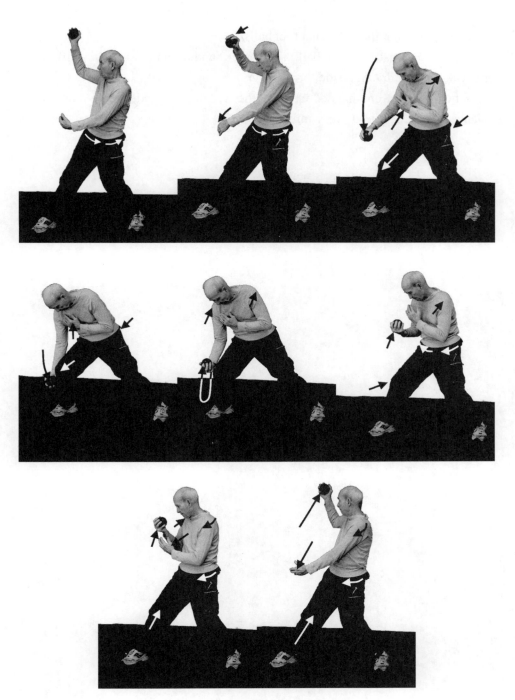

**Figure 66: Bear uproots tree.**

Repeat without the ball (phantom ball).

Try the exercise with the ball in the other hand (phantom ball as well) to feel or check the withdrawing side.

Since this is a one-handed exercise the withdrawing side usage required for balanced biomechanics is very informative.

## Lu Wen Wei Freestyle

Start by executing the exercises with a step forward at each exercise segment, changing hands at the end of each segment. Initiate the steps with synchronous finger and toe movement. Be aware of your foot plant, centers, and the mother line extensions to your hands and feet. Try Bear Uproots Trees alternating hands at each stance position.

When this is familiar and you sustain a good flow with the exercises, combine the three Lu Wen Wei exercises with each other. Randomly move from exercise to exercise, interspersing figure-8s, circles, stepping, etc. For example, as you finish the move into a back stance in pouncing tiger, execute a bear uproots trees and merge back into pouncing tiger.

I particularly liked this moving in and out of the Bear Uproots Trees exercise. One can be interspersed at almost any point using large or small figure-8s.

Then work with a phantom ball; then with punches, keeping the feeling of the ball and eventually adding in some front kicks.

Be sure to do this with the ball in the other (withdrawing side) hand. This is excellent for internalizing, empty arm technique, etc.

Once the above freestyle combining is familiar, work in critical edge maneuvering and flow and/or other concepts of interest. Remember to keep the mind just ahead of the ball. Also work with a visualized ball in the pelvic cup.

Then, without the ball, move to pure shadow boxing with visualized opponents; maintain the same "feeling" you had with the foregoing exercises. With the exception of sparring I found this to be the best vehicle for exploration of integration of the three body systems.

## *Other Exercises*

### Pulling Chi Exercise

After becoming familiar with the above three ball exercises, anyone becoming interested in the internal aspects of the martial arts may find this exercise a good place to start. After these are familiar, perform the three ball exercises blended with the chi pulling material.

Pulling Chi is a translation of La Chi, which is also known as Siphoning Chi.

The hands are the logical starting point for an exercise to study pulling chi. They are the most sensitive and dexterous of the extremities. Consider the chi gates on page 57 and William C.C. Chen's reference to initiation as quoted on page 54, where he states, "The fingers [act] to move palms and fists, and body follows." I think that successful pulling chi exercises for the hands and possibly feet would result in a superior execution of whole-body movements and enhanced mobility.

The prerequisites are the usual: relaxation, breathing, and other Tai Chi conditions. Additionally, you should have a distraction-free environment so you will be able to focus on the exercise.

#### Stage One

1. Sit in a chair with your hands on your thighs, palms down.
2. Close your eyes and focus your attention on your hands.
3. Put your attention or intent (Yi) on the base of the palms.
4. Move your attention to the fingertips.
5. Continue moving the attention between the palms and the fingertips for at least 10 cycles, though 15 are optimal.

The expected primary result is the sensation of movement between base of the palms and the fingertips. A secondary result will be the sensation of "filling" in the hands. Note that you can focus on only one hand if that makes it easier.

### Stage Two

Put your hands in various positions, e.g., thumbs up, thumbs out, and do the same exercise. When this drill is successful, then stand up in the ready position and do the exercises with the arms in the usual "holding ball" position, varying the hand positions, e.g., palms facing up, in, down, out, etc. Also use various palm heights and distances: as high as the eyes, as low as the pelvis, close to the body, and with arms extended (but not straight or locked). In Stage Two, first do the exercises with the eyes closed and then with the eyes open.

### Stage Three

Find the exercises that work best for you and use your eyes to assist in moving by directing your gaze to your palm base and fingertips as your mental focus shifts between them. Use both hands but look only at one hand.

There are variations in moving the chi. For example, circle the chi around the hands by focusing on the individual fingertips in succession, starting with the index finger and then in a circle around the palm to the thumb, or between thumb and forefinger, etc.

### Stage Four

Standing in a high horse stance or ready position move the intent/chi from the palms to the elbows and then back to the palms, making multiple cycles. Be sure you are relaxed and in agreement with gravity, i.e. no local tension in the musculature. The sensation you will experience will be the movement of the body front and back when the intent goes from hands to elbows and back, and then from side to side when the intent alternates between the hands.

This is a good set of drills to transition from pumping the chi from the tantien to siphoning the chi from the tantien and in moving the chi throughout the body. Using these drills as a practical basis, one can learn to pull or siphon chi to various body parts. This set of drills was suggested by my brother Curt as a practical demonstration of the relative ease of experiencing a very basic level of the intentional control of chi.

As always, if you are the experimental type of practitioner, DO NOT MOVE CHI TO THE HEAD IN CHI GONG EXERCISES unless you have the guidance of an experienced instructor! At most, pull the chi to the neck but no further.

## Stepping

In bio-mechanically correct walking the hips are always "in" and the body moves along in a very balanced manner as shown.

There are several other ways to step in combat but this is the most natural and probably the easiest to use for starting with the ball practice. Notice how the opposite shoulder and knee move similarly across the intersection of the hips. Notice how the torso coils and recoils as you move along. The muscles that manage and balance the coiling action of the opposite hip and shoulder as you move are mainly the outer core external oblique, the internal oblique, and the transverse abdominus.

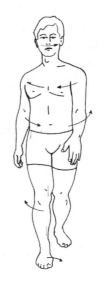

**Figure 67: Counter-rotation during biomechanically correct walking.**

The boxing right cross and the reverse punch of Japanese karate derive much of their upper body force from this coiling action although it must be noted that those techniques also involve spiraling torso contractions involving the latissimus dorsi, serratus anterior, intercostals, and other upper body muscles.

The upper body model for fist strikes one sometimes encounters, where the whole body is depicted as one solid unit that is rotated from the hips toward the opponent, is relatively ineffective. The above-cited muscles plus the inner core multifidus and even the tiny rototores have important roles to play if maximum integration and power potential is to be realized. These latter core muscles run with the spinal column/mother line complex.

All these muscles wrap the body, and maximum force application is usually achieved by spirals in a twisting motion much like the commonly applied twisting down of the thumb side of the fist by the forearm muscles in a straight punch or a boxer's left hook. As you progress in the practice below to become more combat-like, these other muscles increasingly come into play.

Walk around until you feel that you are moving in accordance with the pictures in Figure 69 and Figure 70.

Walk with the hands describing a figure-8 pattern of movement. Use very small hand movements at first. Gradually increase the size of the pattern, being careful to maintain the coordination of hand and foot motion. There should be no sensation of local strength, for example in the shoulder or bicep. Remember to include the feet and hands as initiators.

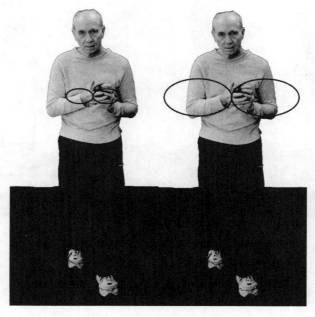

**Figure 68: Walking with figure-8 patterns of the ball.**

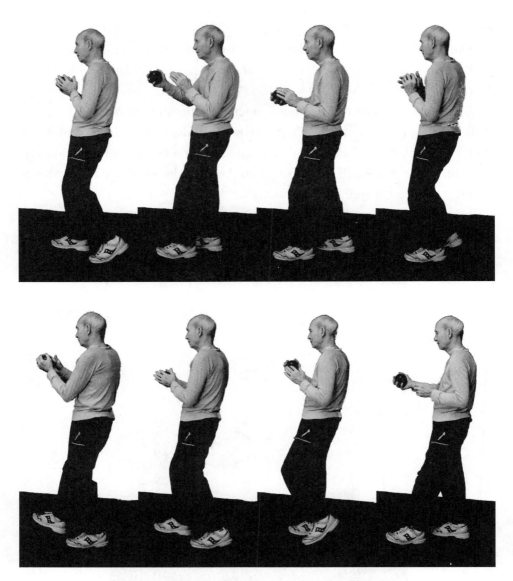

**Figure 69: Walking with the ball (side view).**

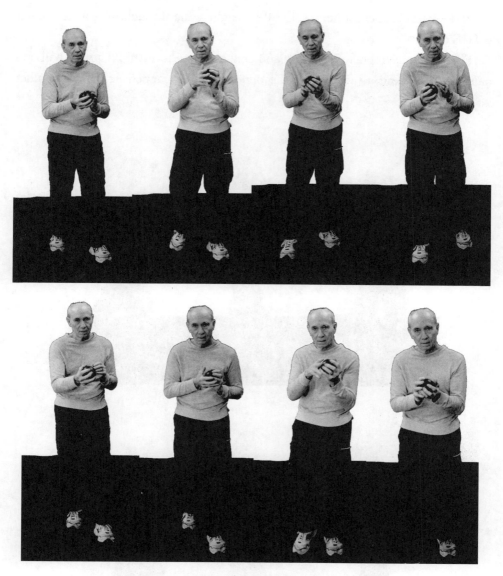

**Figure 70: Walking with the ball (front view).**

Move around as shown, gradually increasing the pace and vigor of the motion. Work to feel that the hands, feet, and centers are moving the ball and the body in a constant flow while focused and aligned on a visualized opponent directly in front of you. Be sure you don't let the shoulders rise up or tension creep into the neck and shoulders. Breathing should be smooth and unforced.

Hold the ball at chest height. Let the weight settle through the middle center to THE center.

Feel the adjustments your body and centers make to manipulate the ball and maintain focus and alignment on the opponent. The cupped pelvis ball holder

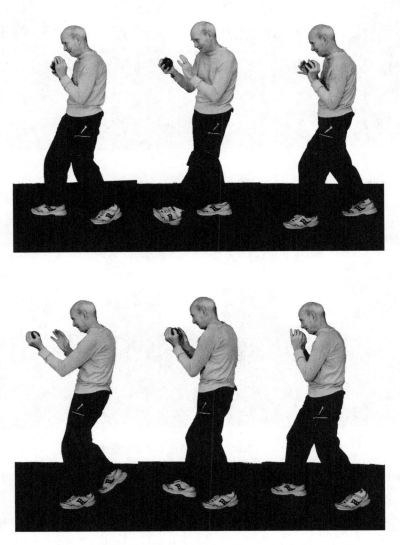

**Figure 71: Walking forward with a straight punch.**

visualization is useful here. Begin transferring the ball from hand to hand with each step (the ball is closely following the visualized opponent) while maintaining the natural form of the illustration.

Note that you walk forward while matching the ball's movement to that of the legs as before. The ball moves in the pattern as shown and the empty hand is in front of the chest until it moves to receive the ball.

Orient the hands in the same manner as in the Lu Wen Wei exercises. Apply the withdrawing side feeling you used in Lu's exercises.

Extend the movement of the ball until you are modeling a straight punch, which flows seamlessly into a return to the chest for a transfer to the other hand.

Work to feel the hands, feet, and centers moving the ball and executing the continuous attacks. Feel the ready rotations of the middle center "ball" and work to develop an awareness of the mother line connection of the centers as you move and execute the attacks. If you have not already done so, this is a good place to begin visualizing mother line extensions to the hands and feet if you wish to use that model and to use hands and feet as initiators.

- - -

Hold the ball a bit lower in front of the chest.

Start walking forward in a balanced way as before while raising the ball up in an uppercut as shown in Figure 72.

Again the ball is retracted seamlessly back and down to be transferred to the other hand. Feel the centers moving the ball. The middle center ball rotations can be applied at varying angles to vary attack angle (elbow action is important here). Feel the mother line and its extensions working.

**Combine stepping and side to side, add turning.**

Visualize the opponent retreating in front of you in a backward weaving pattern. Follow, thrusting with the ball in the various punches practiced above. Add turns and pivots. Work in defensive techniques: blocks, counters, and then add in the occasional kick. Maintain the elements cited above, tactile hands with the ball, the active resilient feet, dynamic centers (with knees), critical edge, etc.

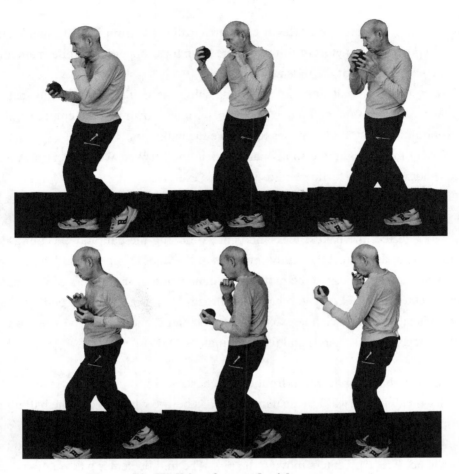

**Figure 72: Walking forward with an uppercut.**

Repeat the above process without the ball but using real clenched fist techniques. Morph into real shadow boxing; be sure to include your offensive and defensive combat techniques. Go back and forth between the two methods.

## A Proven Combat Move

This move was originally shown to me many years ago by Harold Gunns, a wonderful boxing teacher. It was used when an opponent was maneuvering aggressively right at you and was quite effective then and has been effective ever since when sparring in various formats. With the ball it is very instructional.

Hold the ball as shown in front of you at chest/throat height. Soften your body. Visualize an opponent closing, extend the ball in the "jab" as shown in Figure 73 without any foot movement.

Just as you begin the ball retraction (which ends with a shift of the ball to the back hand), skip back with the rear leg as shown. Ball retraction and backward shift are simultaneous. Feel the weight of your body and the returning ball (now in the rear hand) settle into your softened body's centers, rear leg, and foot, compressing them. Bounce off this compression into an expansion forward with a ball "cross" and a simultaneous short extension forward with the front leg (which can be left just a bit behind during the backwards shift for a good critical-edge, frontal-weight bias).

Generally, but depending on the distance, the punch can start fractionally before the forward expansion. If the opponent is very close, the ball punch can be started just before the backward skip/compression finishes. In actual sparring, timing and placement of the initial jab is critical. This move works very nicely into the Lu Wen Wei freestyle maneuvers.

This is a very basic example of contraction-expansion. It is also a basic illustration of "spring" energy, a fundamental concept of some styles. There are many applications of these concepts in the forms below. Note that these drills are for right-handed fighters. You should practice left handed as well.

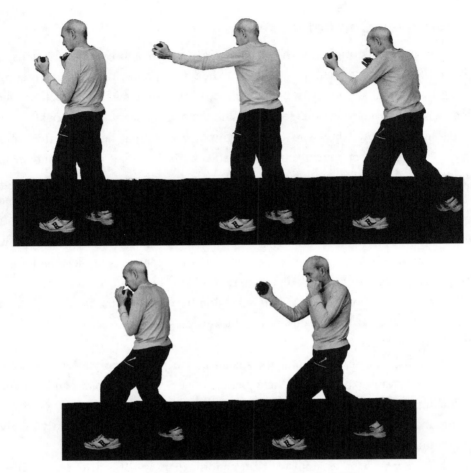

**Figure 73: Combat move with the ball.**

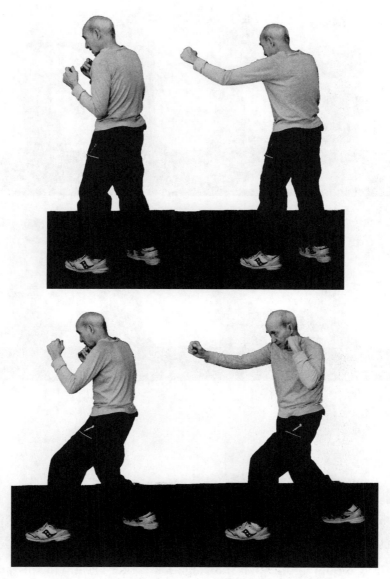

**Figure 74: Application of combat move without the ball. The four pictures show the ready posture, jab without moving feet, retract the jab while skipping back, and fire the cross the instant the back foot lands.**

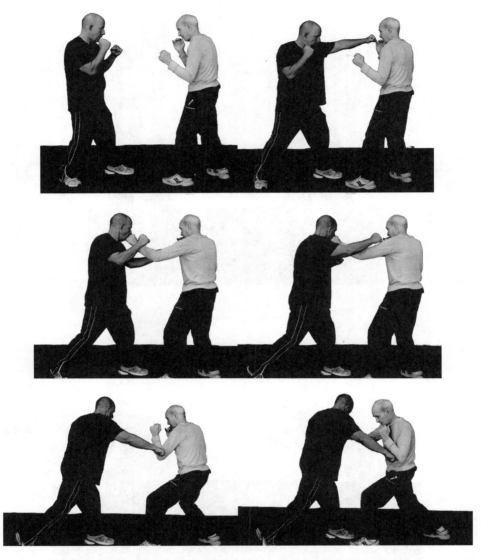

**Figure 75: Combat application showing an attacker closing the distance with a left jab as the defender fades slightly back. The defender jabs just as the attacker begins his follow-up right cross and steps back a bit with the retraction of his jab. The defender compresses his body (legs, centers, feet, etc.) then seamlessly flows into a full body expansion into the attacker's follow-on momentum. See page 137 for additional details of this technique.**

# 4. The Forms

There are four forms here: the staff, ball, phantom ball, and empty hand forms. The staff form is the template, taken from Wan Lai Sheng's book. I wanted to apply the very positive results I had felt from working with the ball to weapons and empty hands practice. The staff form is short and quite dynamic. It has excellent transitioning sequences, reasonably challenging moves, and provides rather unique value in developing expansion/contraction plus withdrawing side and other internalizing abilities. I felt that the contrast between the four basically identical forms would provide good insight into the principles and concepts I had been struggling with for a long time.

Note that the forms are not identical. The ball is a training tool, not a weapon. Exactly replicating weapons or weaponless strikes and blocks with the ball is awkward, if not impossible. I made some changes (including different combinations of movements 9-12 in the staff form for the ball and empty-hands forms). The goal was to preserve a good flow and maintain the same challenges to critical-edge mobility, whole-body movement, good structure, etc. This is the whole objective and so far it has provided some pretty decent insights.

The order is not fixed. Feel free to experiment. If a change would be a better approach to your own main interests, style-based emphasis, or problems, make it. For example, the phantom ball form below is a recent addition based on ideas generated with training partners. The basic staff form is very well suited to experimentation. I do feel that its excellent flow with structural variety in maneuver are its strong points, but, for example, with an eye to internalizing/withdrawing study, I added circles after some of the thrusts in the ball version of the form. This was like multiple hooking off a jab and was a good variation to practice. After training recently with Pat Strong, I became more interested in disruptive techniques and inserted some in each of the versions where they

141

seemed logical. This was all quite interesting, but I feel that such experimentation should come well after the basic structure, flow, and maneuver concepts are well integrated. The questions inherent in studying the center model, critical edge, mother line, foot plant, and the rest are tough enough without adding additional complications.

## Balancing the Forms

Forms such as the Sil Lum Dao of the Wing Chun style are "balanced" in that they are executed exactly the same on the right and left side. Other styles such as the Japanese and Okinawan seem to be mainly right handed although the Gankaku Den form does have a definite left-hand bias. The Tekki (Naihanchi) forms show good balance.

Since this staff form, like so many, is "right handed," executing it "left handed" is a good idea. It is a short form so this is relatively easy to do. Doing the most complex parts first then moving to the whole sequence when they feel natural seems to work fairly well. "If you can only fight on one side, you are only half a fighter" is a saying that has some validity. For an obvious example, if someone wanted to make a surprise attack on you, they would be on statistically solid ground if they casually came up on your right side and launched their assault. You would be fighting as a "lefty." Of course this logic does not apply if you are Bruce-Lee-style trained (strong/right side forward).

## Chinese Staff Form

This form is executed in a continuous flow. Note that the illustrations are not a series of poses or focal points but rather are movements that are seamlessly passed through.

When executing the forms, your eyes should be focused at the point in space where the opponent would be. Do not focus out ahead of you into infinity. This applies to any practice of basics or drills as well. Your peripheral vision close to you will be affected. It is an unrealistic habit to develop. Do not go there.

The length of the staff is a matter of personal preference. You do see some very long tapered staffs about eight feet long and also some short four-foot staffs. The longest basic staff I have heard of would reach from the ground to the palm of a person's hand extended straight overhead. The Japanese staff is about six feet long. In Wan Lai Sheng's book the staff length is given as reaching from the ground to the eyebrows. All lengths should be experimented with. The longer staffs require more strength and room to maneuver. This could be a handicap in closer quarters or in a crowded melee. The pictures of the eyebrow level staff from the old Wan Lai Shen book show a more versatile movement capability. This has been my own experience in our low ceiling training hall, but outside in an open space I have to maneuver really well to maintain equality with the longer staffs.

When executing techniques with the staff, pay attention to the pulling/ withdrawing side. Force is generated with the whole body from the feet to the hands with a balanced withdrawing side and striking side. The force moves around the mother line for the most part. If one side has some emphasis, it is usually the withdrawing side. In other words, the rear hand is the power hand and the front hand is the targeting hand. There are several fan to zan and zan to fan transitions here, work to make them fluid, dynamic, and seamless.

The foot positions for each of the moves are shown in the ball form.

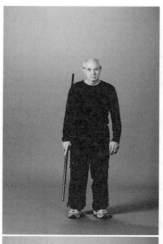
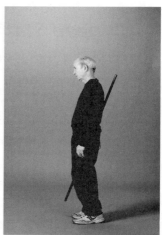

To start the form stand naturally with the staff in your right hand. The right hand grips the staff at the upper third.

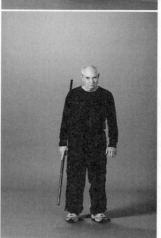
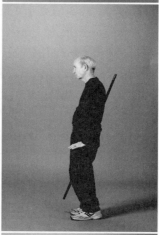

1. Assume the combat posture. Consider critical edge, tilted pelvis, softened chest, widened back, bubbling well, awareness of the centers, etc. Awareness extends in all directions. See, feel, and hear the room. The hands are at the sides with the left-hand palm facing the floor and the staff is held inverted and parallel to the body as shown.

2. Step into a ready position, left foot forward. Both hands come up into a guard position. The left hand is open, the staff is held along the right forearm. Weight is about 70% on the rear leg.

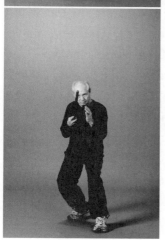
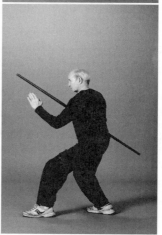

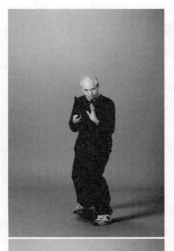

3. Take a short sliding step forward with the left leg.

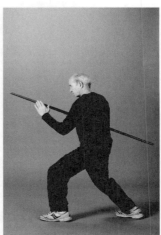

4. Take a full step forward with the right leg.

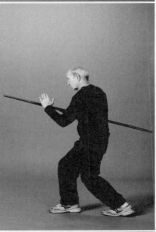

5. Take a full step forward with the left leg. During these first movements the feeling is of awareness in all directions while smoothly and carefully walking forward.

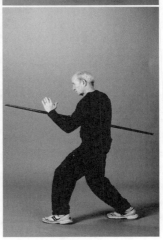

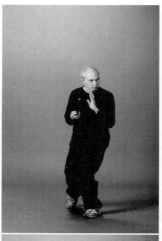

6. Step forward with the right leg, simultaneously gripping the staff with the left hand at the bottom third and looking to the left. Shift your awareness more strongly to the left where the major opponent is but retain some focus on the sides and rear. Until the end of the form awareness rests primarily with but not completely in the direction of the major threat. Critical edge orientation follows awareness.

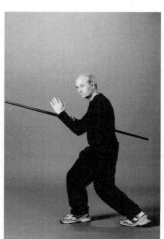

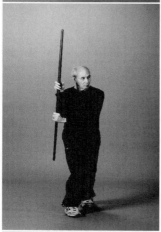

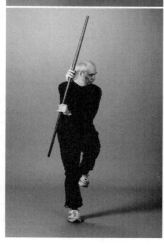

7. Stand up on the right leg with a strong expansive feeling. The right elbow comes to the inside of the staff. The left foot rises dynamically to the left side of the right knee.

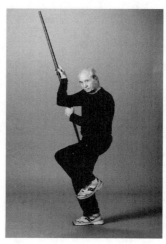

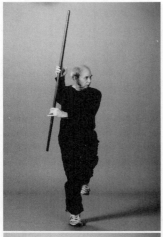

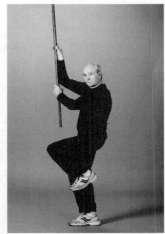

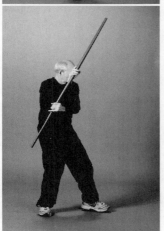

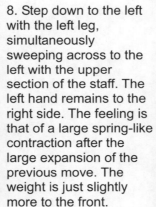

8. Step down to the left with the left leg, simultaneously sweeping across to the left with the upper section of the staff. The left hand remains to the right side. The feeling is that of a large spring-like contraction after the large expansion of the previous move. The weight is just slightly more to the front.

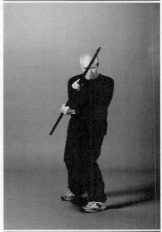

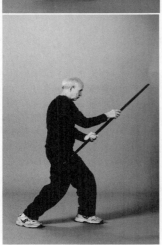

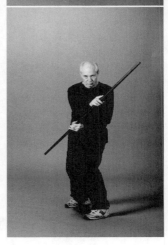

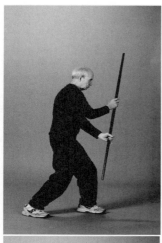

9. The arms continue around, hands switching sides, arcing up into an upper level block. There is a slight feeling of expansion and of getting in with a slight weight shift forward near the end of the block.

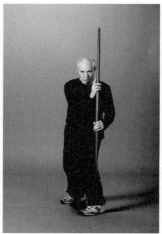

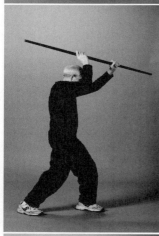

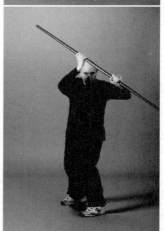

10. Continue the arm motion around and down for a right-hand strike. There should be a feeling of strong contraction and a slight further weight shift forward. Moves 8, 9, and 10 are two blocks against an attack combination and your counter strike.

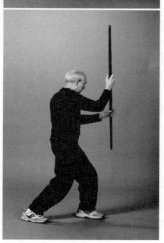

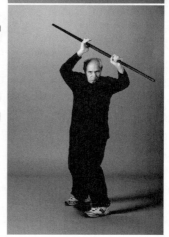

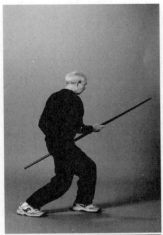

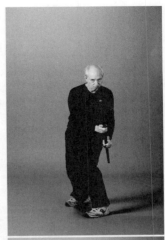

11. Lean forward and to the left while hooking back and to the right with the right hand.

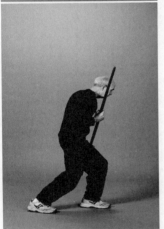

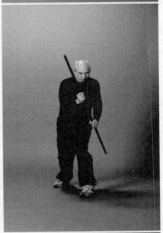

12. Quickly step forward across the left leg with the right leg as shown while turning the body to the right and simultaneously sweeping the staff down across to the right in a lower level block with the left hand. Moves 11 and 12 are done as one motion. The feeling is that of an inwardly coiling contraction.

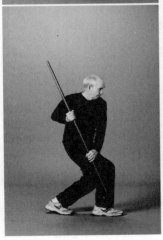

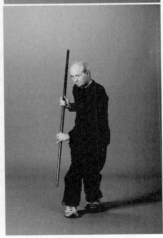

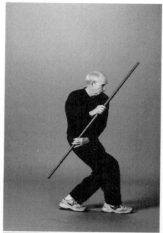

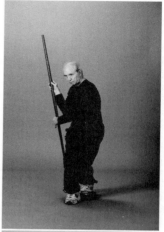

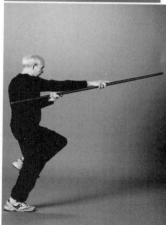

13. Instantly stand up strongly on the right leg, the body uncoiling to the front with a strong feeling of expansion. The staff simultaneously thrusts forward with the right hand, the left hand remains at the right side of the body. The left leg comes up dynamically with the strong right hip movement, with the left foot resting just at the inside knee level.

14. Step down and strongly forward a half step with the left leg.

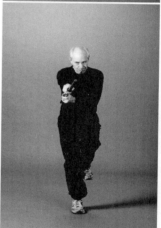

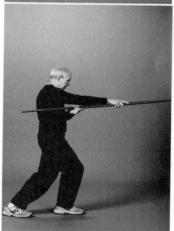

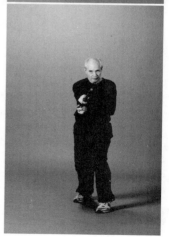

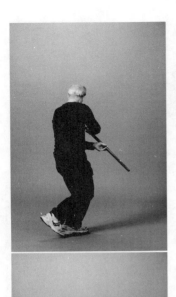

15. Step seamlessly forward with the right leg while turning to the rear and executing an upper level block against an overhead strike. The weight is more on the rear leg.

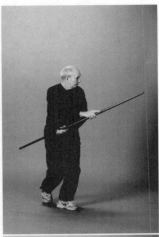

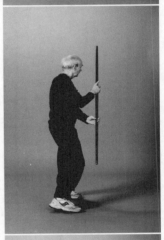

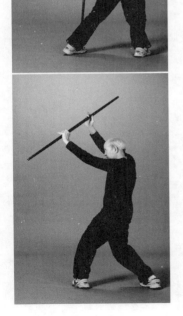

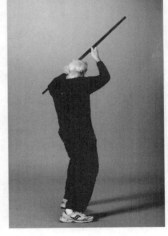

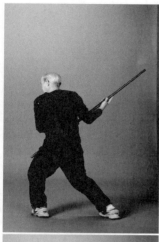

16. Hook back to the right with the staff with a feeling of getting in and a slight weight shift forward.

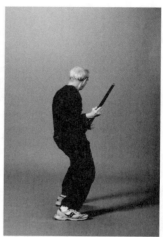

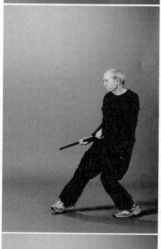

17. Step in deeply with the right leg and strike strongly at the opponent's knee. The hips turn over strongly with the strike. Weight remains mostly on the left leg.

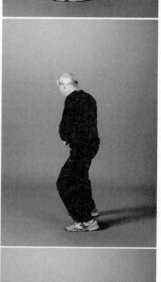

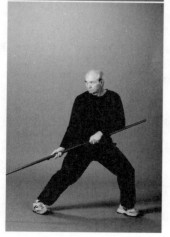

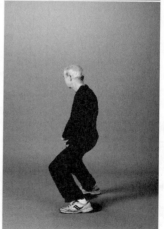

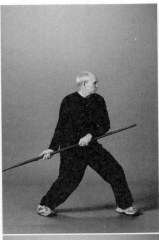

18. Look to the rear and retreat by stepping back behind the right leg with the left leg. At the same time the right hand sweeps the staff across the body from right to left. The left hand swings the lower end of the staff to the right. The body remains faced to the side and the feeling is of strong contraction.

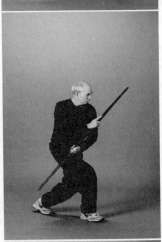

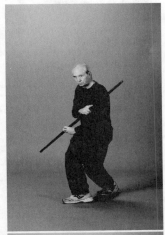

19. Quickly rebound off the contraction of 18 with a strong expansion into a left foot middle level front stamping kick and a simultaneous left-hand upper level thrust with the staff.

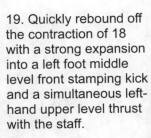

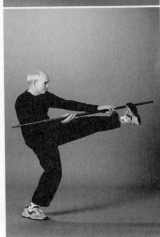

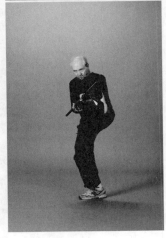

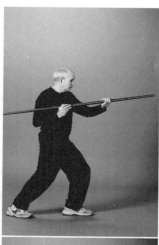

20. Step strongly down to the front with the left foot and then continue on into a step forward with the right leg while executing a right side overhead strike.

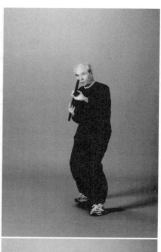

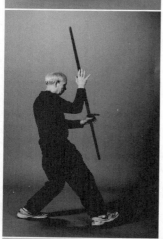

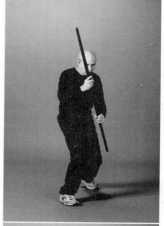

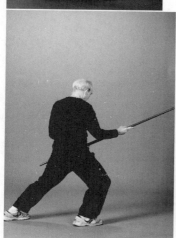

Right view

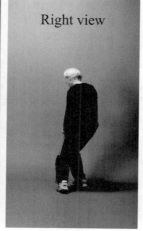

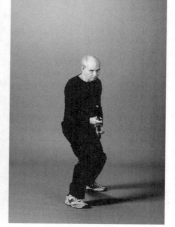

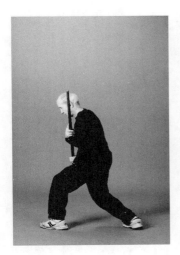

21. Pivot to the rear in place, contracting strongly into a sweeping right-hand block from right to left while coiling down and in. The left hand crosses under to the right side during the move. The body inclines somewhat to the front and the weight is largely on the rear leg.

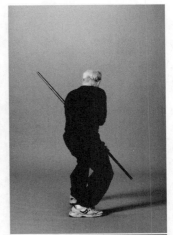

Right view

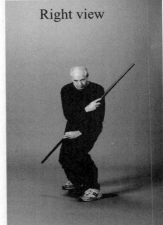

Right view

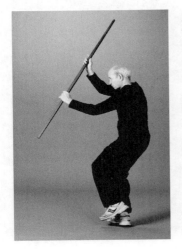

22. Quickly rebound off the contraction, uncoiling expansively up into a "thunder step" (stamp). The right foot stomps down loudly (like thunder) next to the left foot while the staff executes a thrusting block in and up to unbalance the opponent. The left leg comes up dynamically with the body. The left foot is at the right knee.

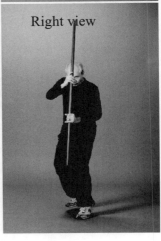

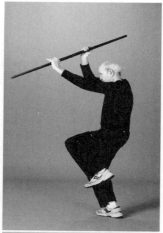

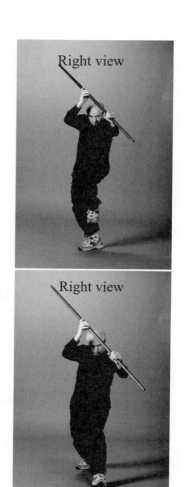

23. Step strongly down and to the front with the left leg and continue on into a step forward with the right leg while executing a right side overhead strike.

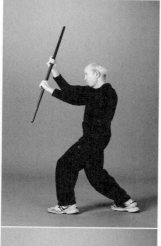

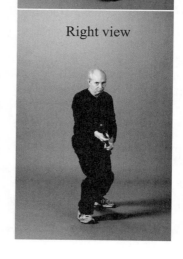

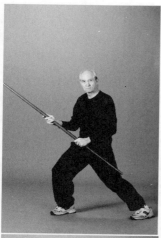

Return to the upright combat posture.

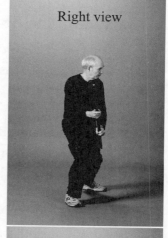

Right view

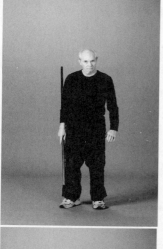

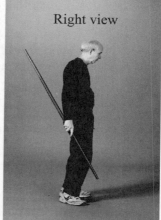

Right view

Assume a natural stance.

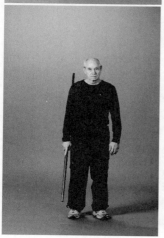

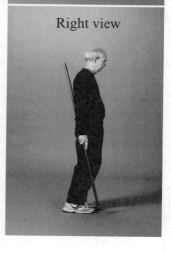

Right view

## Balancing the Staff Form

L7. Stand up on the left leg. The left hand grips the staff at the top third and the left elbow is on the inside of the staff. The right hand grips the staff at the bottom third and at the left side of the body. The right foot moves to the right side of the left knee. Look to the right.

L8. Step to the right with the right leg, simultaneously sweeping across to the right with the upper section of the staff. The right hand remains at the left side.

L9. The arms continue around, hands switching sides, arcing up into an upper level block.

L10. Continue the arm motion around and down for a left-hand strike.

L11. Lean forward and to the right while hooking back and to the left with the left hand.

L12. Quickly step forward across the right leg with the left leg while turning the body to the left and simultaneously sweeping the staff down across to the left in a lower level block with the right hand.

L13. Instantly stand up strongly on the left leg as the body turns to the front with a strong feeling of expansion. The staff simultaneously thrusts forward with the left hand, the right hand remains at the left side of the body. The right leg comes up dynamically with the strong left hip movement. The right foot is just at the inside knee level.

Raise the staff to vertical, move the left elbow to the inside of the staff, look to the right.

Repeat the L7-L13 sequence until it feels natural, and then move to the next set of techniques.

L16. Stand as at the end of 16 but reversed. The right leg is forward, and the weight is about evenly distributed. The staff is held with the left hand back and the right more to the front, etc.

L17. Step in deeply with the left leg and strike strongly at the opponent's knee.

L18. Look to the rear and retreat by stepping back behind the left leg with the right leg. At the same time the left hand sweeps the staff across the body from left to right. The right hand swings the lower end of the staff to the left. The body remains faced to the side and the feeling is of strong contraction.

L19. Quickly rebound off the contraction of L18 with a strong expansion into a right, middle level, front stamping kick and a simultaneous right-hand upper level thrust with the staff.

L20. Step down strongly to the front with the right foot and then continue on into a step forward with the left leg while executing a left side overhead strike.

Turn to the rear in place. You are now in the approximate posture of L16.

Cycle L16-L20 until they feel natural and then move to the next set of techniques.

L21. Stand in the final position of L20. Pivot to the rear in place contracting strongly into a sweeping left-hand block from left to right while coiling down and in. The right hand crosses under to the left during the move.

L22. Quickly rebound off the contraction, uncoiling expansively up into a "thunder step" while executing a thrusting block in and up to unbalance the opponent. The right leg comes up dynamically with the body. The right foot is at the left knee.

L23. Step strongly down and to the front with the right leg and continue on into a step forward with the left leg while executing a left side overhead strike.

You are now in the posture of the end of L20. Cycle through L21-L23 until they feel natural.

Add in the simpler parts of the form from the beginning. After some repetition the "left-handed" form will begin to feel natural.

## Ball Form

Preparation is the same as for the staff: hips, critical edge, etc. The weight of the ball will add to the feeling going down the side of the body. This will require a counterbalancing increase on the other side. This increased upper body feeling should be met with an increase in feeling from the ground up the inside of the legs, the hips, and buttocks to the spinal column. The intersection of the ascending and descending feelings is that place inside the lower abdomen referred to as THE center, tantien, tanden, etc. Feel that the center of THE center, the pelvic cup, holds the ball.

Be aware of the mother line extension of THE center and the other centers if that is your model. The center/centers and the ball should feel light and mobile.

It might be a good idea to wear shoes. Dropping the ball on your feet is a possibility, especially at first. Shoes offer some protection and, after all, training in a variety of dress is realistic.

Side views of the ball forms can be seen by studying the phantom ball form.

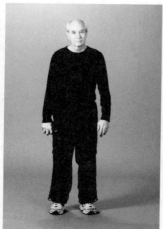

Stand in a natural stance. With the weight of the ball to consider it is worth noting that awareness of the centers and critical-edge maintenance should be a primary concern at the beginning of work on this version of the form.

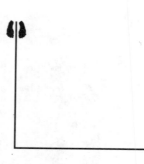

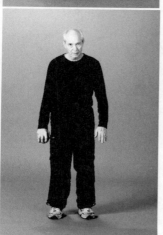

1. Assume the combat posture. Awareness extends in all directions, See, feel, and hear the room. The arms are at the sides, the left palm faces the floor, and the right hand holds the ball as shown.

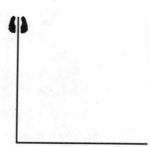

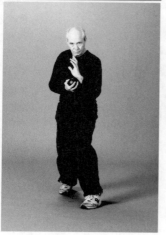

2. Step into a ready position. The left foot is forward. Weight is about 70% on the rear leg. Both hands come up into a guard position. The left hand is open. The right hand and THE center are holding the ball.

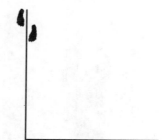

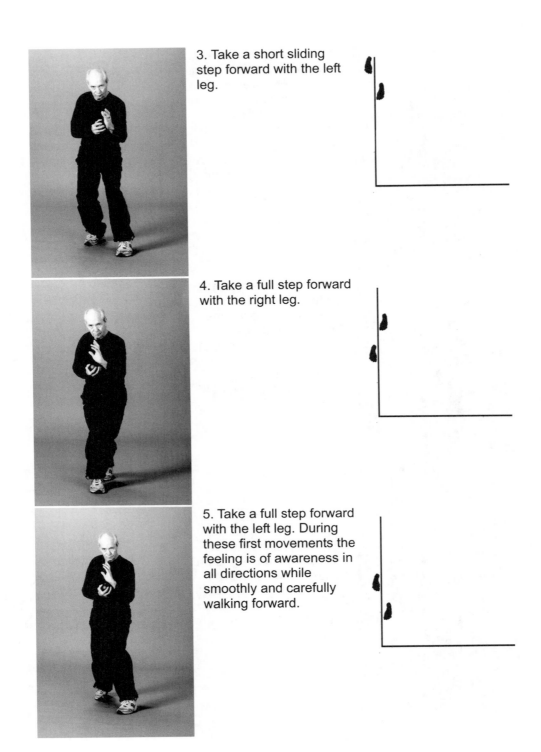

3. Take a short sliding step forward with the left leg.

4. Take a full step forward with the right leg.

5. Take a full step forward with the left leg. During these first movements the feeling is of awareness in all directions while smoothly and carefully walking forward.

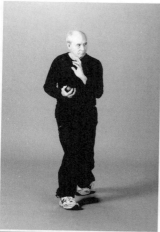

6. Step forward with the right leg simultaneously looking to the left. Shift your awareness more strongly to the left where the major threat is but retain some focus to the sides and rear. Until the end of the form awareness rests primarily but not completely in the direction of the major threat. This is also true of critical edge orientation.

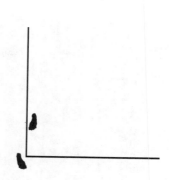

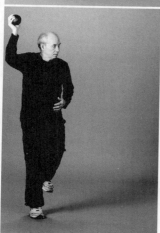

7. Stand up on the right leg with a strong expansive feeling as shown. The hips, left knee, and the ball in the right hand all complete the expansion simultaneously. The left foot rests at the inside of the right knee. The left hand may be positioned in a guard position in front of the sternum to match the staff version or it may make a lower level block.

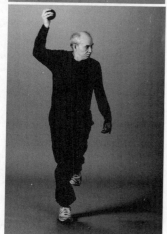

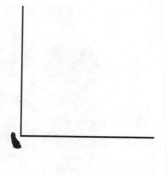

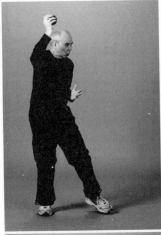

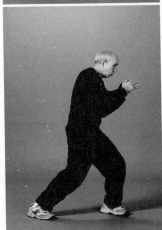

8. Step down to the left with the left leg, simultaneously sweeping down and out a bit to the front with both hands and just slightly across to the left. The hands having extended out then come back in slightly while shifting the ball to the left hand. The feeling is that of a large spring-like contraction after the previous move's expansion. The weight is just slightly to the front side.

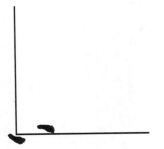

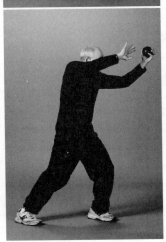

9-10. Flow into an expansion striking out to the upper level with the ball in the left hand while simultaneously executing an upper level block with the right arm. There is a feeling of getting in with the double-hand movement.

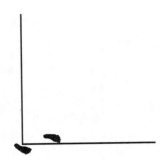

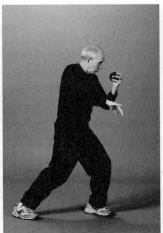

11. Retract back from the double move in preparation for stepping forward.

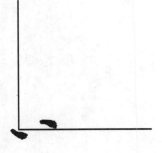

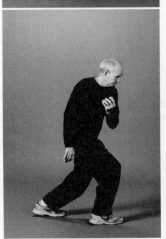

12. Both hands pull strongly back with the body turning forcefully to the right while the right leg simultaneously steps forward across the left leg. The left hand with the ball sweeps back across to the right at shoulder level while the right hand sweeps back down across at knee level. The feeling is that of coiling in and somewhat down.

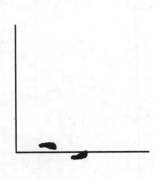

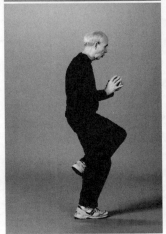

13. Seamlessly stand up strongly on the right leg, the body uncoils to the front with a strong feeling of expansion. As the body uncoils to the front, the ball transfers to the right hand, which thrusts the ball forward at face level. The left hand comes to the guard position or makes a pulling hand, as shown. The left leg comes up dynamically with the strong right hip

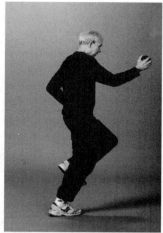

movement. The left foot is just at the inside right knee level.

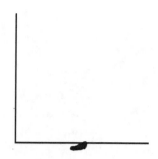

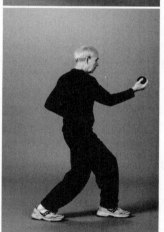

14. Step down and strongly forward a half step with the left leg. Awareness shifts to the rear.

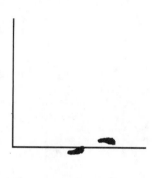

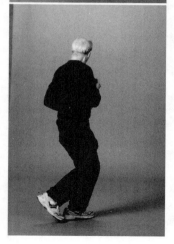

15. Step forward with the right leg while turning to the rear and executing a double upper level block as shown. During the turn the ball has transferred to the left hand. The weight is more to the rear leg.

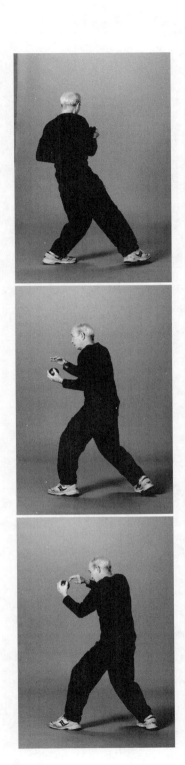

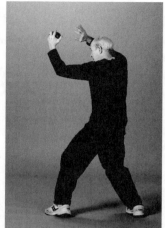

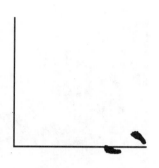

16. Sweep both hands back to shoulder level as shown with a feeling of getting in and a slight weight shift forward.

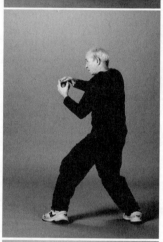

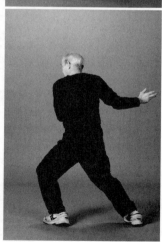

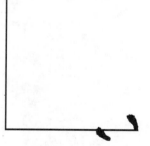

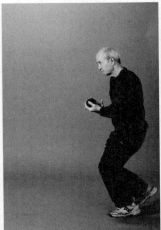

17. Step in deeply with the right leg as shown. At the beginning of the step the ball has transferred to the right hand and then strikes at the tantien level. The left hand is at the guard position in front of the chest. The strike can also be done at the rib level.

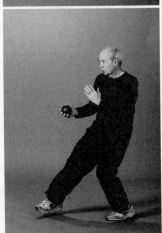

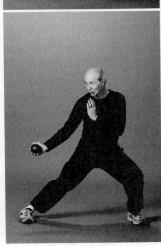

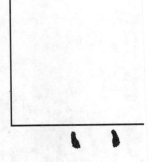

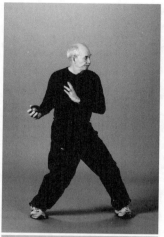

18. Look to the rear and step back and behind the right leg with the left leg. At the same time the right hand sweeps the ball across the body from right to left. The left hand moves with the right hand. The body remains faced to the side and the feeling is of strong contraction.

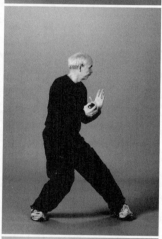

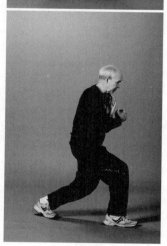

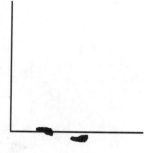

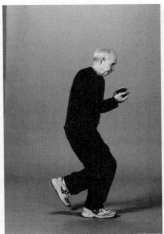

19. Seamlessly rebound off the contraction with a strong expansion into a left front stamping kick at diaphragm level and a simultaneous left-hand upper level thrust with the ball, which has transferred from the right hand at the beginning of the expansion.

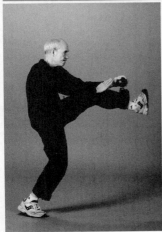

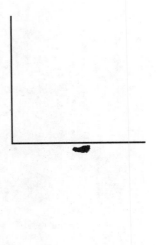

20. Step strongly down to the front with the left foot while retracting back and transferring the ball to the right hand. Continue seamlessly on into a step forward with the right leg while thrusting to the upper level with the ball.

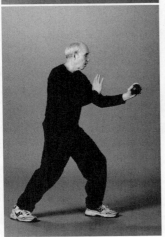

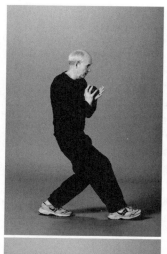

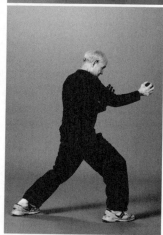

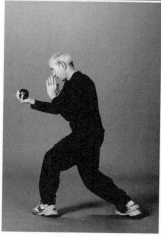

21. Pivot to the rear in place, contracting strongly down into a sweeping right-hand middle level forearm block while coiling down and in. The left hand comes around to the guard position as shown. The body is inclined somewhat to the front and the weight is largely on the rear leg.

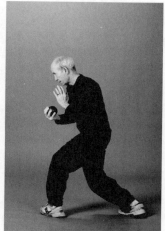

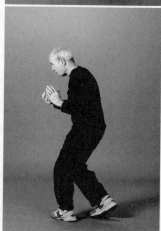

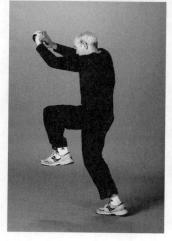

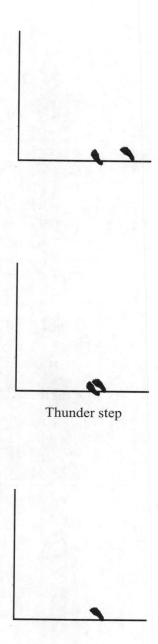

22. Seamlessly rebound off the contraction, uncoiling expansively up into a "thunder step" (stamp). The right foot moves next to the left foot stamping strongly down with a noise like thunder while both arms execute a thrusting block up and in to unbalance the opponent. The ball is transferred to the left hand just at the beginning of the movement. The left leg comes up dynamically with the body. The left foot is at the inside of the right knee.

There is an extremely quick weight shift back and forth required here between movements 21 and 22 if a successful one-motion number 22 is to be performed. It is a good study of the role of the feet.

Thunder step

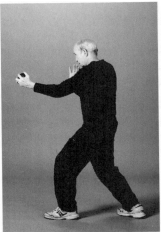

23. Step strongly down and to the front with the left leg while retracting the hands back and transferring the ball to the right hand. Continue seamlessly on into a step forward with the right leg while executing an upper level thrust with the ball.

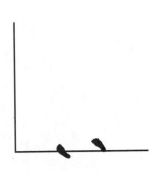

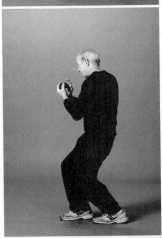

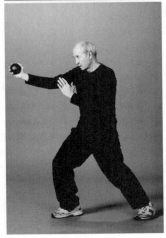

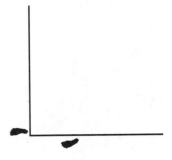

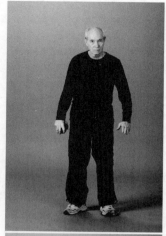

Return to the upright
combat posture.

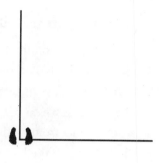

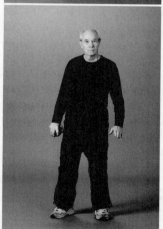

Assume a natural stance.

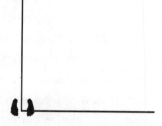

## Balancing the Ball Form

L7. Stand up on the left leg. The right foot rests at the inside of the left knee. Look to the right. The right hand is in a guard position in front of the sternum. The ball is held overhead in the left hand

L8. Step down to the right with the right leg, simultaneously sweeping down and out to the front with both hands and just slightly across to the right. The hands retract and the ball shifts to the right hand.

L9-L10. Flow into an expansion striking out to the upper level with the ball in the right hand while simultaneously executing an upper level block with the left arm.

L11-L12. Both hands pull strongly back with the body turning strongly to the left while the left leg simultaneously steps forward across the right leg. The right hand with the ball sweeps across to the left at shoulder level while the left hand sweeps down across at knee level.

L13. Stand up strongly on the left leg, the body uncoiling to the front. At the beginning of this movement the ball transfers to the left hand, which thrusts the ball forward at face level. The right hand comes to the guard position or pulling hand. The right leg comes up dynamically with the strong left hip movement. The right foot is at the inside left knee level.

Look to the right and raise the ball overhead. Repeat L7 through L13 until it feels natural and then move to the next set of techniques.

L16. Stand in the position at the end of move 16 with the right foot forward and the left foot back. The ball is in the right hand.

L17. Step in deeply with the left leg. At the beginning of the step the ball transfers to the left hand and then strikes at the tantien level. The right hand is in the guard position in front of the chest.

L18. Look to the rear and step back and behind the left leg with the right leg. At the same time the left hand sweeps the ball across the body from left to right. The right hand moves with the left hand. The body remains faced to the side and the feeling is of strong contraction.

L19. Quickly rebound off the contraction with strong expansion into a right front stamping kick at diaphragm level and a simultaneous right-hand upper level thrust with the ball, which has transferred from the left hand at the beginning of the expansion.

L20. Step strongly down to the front with the right foot retracting back and transferring the ball to the left hand. Continue seamlessly on into a step forward with the left leg while thrusting to the upper level with the ball.

You are now in the approximate position of the end of L16. Look to the rear and repeat L16 through L20 until they feel natural then move to the final set of techniques.

L21. Stand in the final position of L20. Then pivot to the rear in place contracting strongly down into a sweeping left-hand forearm block while coiling down and in. The right hand comes around to the guard position. The body inclines somewhat to the front and the weight is largely on the rear leg.

L22. Quickly rebound off the contraction, uncoiling expansively up into a "thunder step" (stamp) with the left leg while executing a thrusting block in and up with both arms to unbalance the opponent. The ball is transferred to the right hand just at the beginning of the movement. The right leg comes up dynamically with the body. The right foot is at the left knee.

L23. Step strongly down and to the front with the right leg retracting back and transferring the ball to the left hand. Continue seamlessly on into a step forward with the left leg while executing an upper level thrust with the ball.

Repeat L21 through L23 until they feel natural. Then add in the simpler parts to the form and do the form from the beginning. After some repetition the whole form will feel natural.

## Phantom Ball Form

Execute the form without the ball while feeling the ball or some energy there in its place. I have found that executing the form slowly in the manner of the Tai Chi practitioners is a very valuable exercise.

Without the ball but with the tactile sense or energy of the hands/fingers felt in coordination with the tactile foot there is a qualitative difference in connecting to the center/centers for a very mobile whole-body feeling. It is also easier to sense the mother line and the pelvic cup visualizations, thereby enhancing the feet, hands, and centers integration. Breath integration is also easy to work into the whole-body feeling with this practice.

Various speeds of execution can, of course, be used, but I feel that the slower execution provides more insight with the phantom ball form.

An informative workout is to cycle through Lu Wen Wei's exercises with the ball, the ball form, and the phantom ball form, occasionally varying the progression.

The foot positions for each of the moves are shown in the ball form.

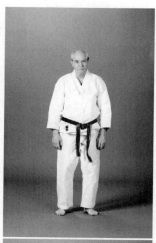

Stand in a natural stance.

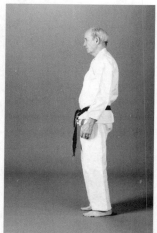

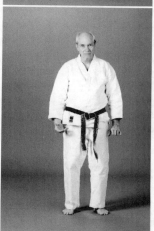

1. Assume the combat posture. Awareness extends in all directions. See, feel, and hear the room. The arms are at the sides, the left palm faces the floor, and the right hand holds the phantom ball as shown.

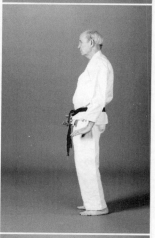

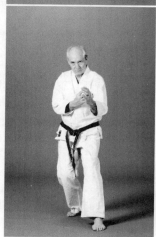

2. Step into a ready position. The left foot is forward. Weight is about 70% on the rear leg. Both hands come up into a guard position. The left hand is open. The right hand and THE center are holding the phantom ball. The presence of a phantom ball means that awareness of the centers and critical-edge maintenance should be a primary concern in this form.

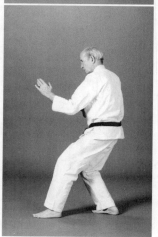

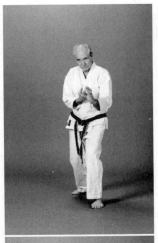

3. Take a short sliding step forward with the left leg.

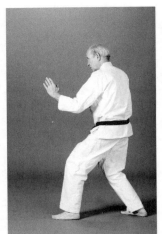

4. Take a full step forward with the right leg.

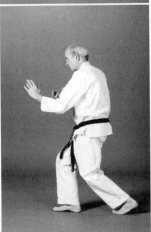

5. Take a full step forward with the left leg. During these first movements the feeling is of awareness in all directions while smoothly and carefully walking forward.

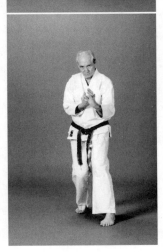

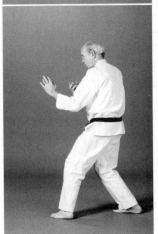

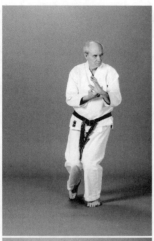

6. Step forward with the right leg simultaneously looking to the left. Shift your awareness more strongly to the left where the major threat is but retain some focus to the sides and rear. Until the end of the form awareness rests primarily but not completely in the direction of the major threat. This is also true of critical edge orientation.

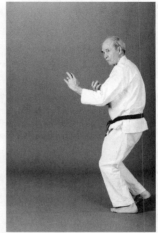

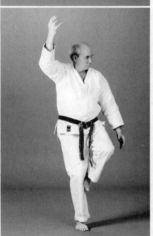

7. Stand up on the right leg with a strong expansive feeling as shown. The hips, left knee and the phantom ball in the right hand all complete the expansion simultaneously. The left foot rests at the inside of the right knee. The left hand makes a lower level block. The left hand may also be positioned in a guard position in front of the sternum.

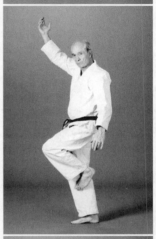

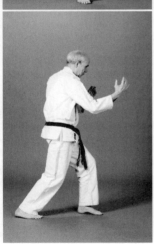

8. Step down to the left with the left leg, simultaneously sweeping down and out a bit to the front with both hands and just slightly across to the left. The hands extend out then come back in slightly while shifting the phantom ball to the left hand. The feeling is that of a large spring-like contraction after the previous move's expansion. The weight is just slightly to the front side.

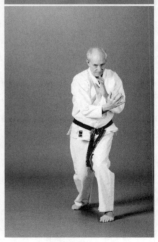

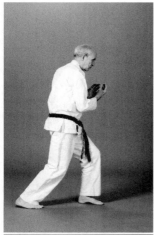

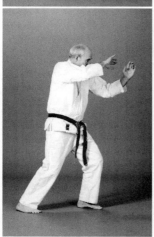

9-10. Flow into an expansion striking out to the upper level with the phantom ball in the left hand while simultaneously executing an upper level block with the right arm. There is a feeling of getting in with the double-hand movement.

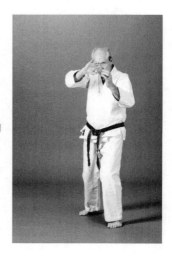

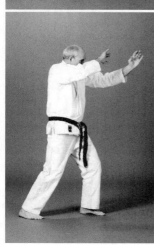

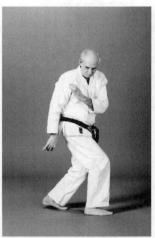

11-12. Both hands pull strongly back with the body turning forcefully to the right while the right leg simultaneously steps forward across the left leg. The left hand with the phantom ball sweeps back across to the right at shoulder level while the right hand sweeps back down across at knee level. The feeling is that of coiling in and somewhat down.

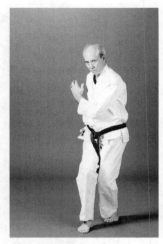

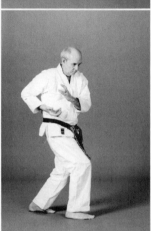

13. Seamlessly stand up strongly on the right leg, the body uncoils to the front with a strong feeling of expansion. As the body uncoils to the front, the phantom ball transfers to the right hand, which thrusts the phantom ball forward at face level. The left hand becomes a pulling hand on the hip or moves to the guard position. The left leg comes up dynamically with the strong right hip movement. The left foot is just at the inside right knee level.

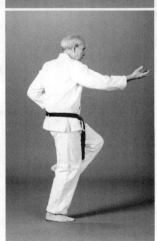

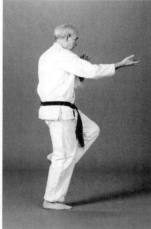

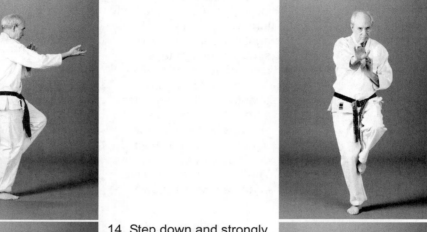

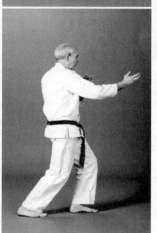

14. Step down and strongly forward a half step with the left leg. Awareness shifts to the rear.

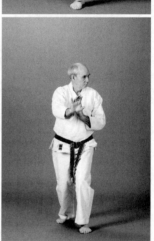

15. Step forward with the right leg while turning to the rear and executing a double upper level block as shown. During the turn the phantom ball has transferred to the left hand. The weight is more on the rear leg.

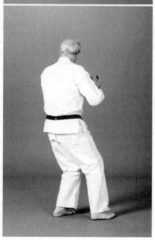

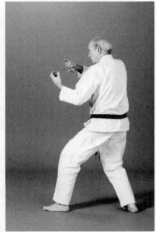

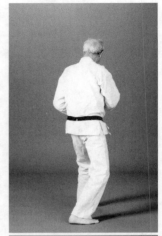

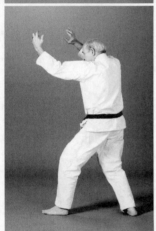

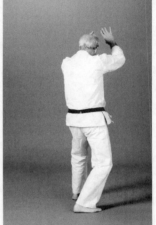

16. Sweep both hands back to shoulder level as shown with a feeling of getting in and a slight weight shift forward.

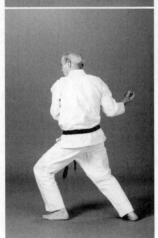

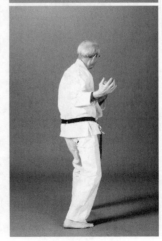

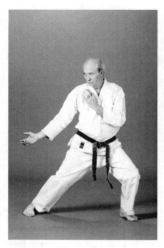

17. Step in deeply with the right leg as shown. At the beginning of the step the phantom ball has transferred to the right hand and then strikes at tantien level. The left hand is at the guard position in front of the chest.

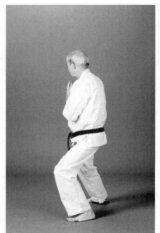

18. Look to the rear and step back and behind the right leg with the left leg. At the same time the right hand sweeps the phantom ball across the body at face level from right to left. The left hand moves with the right hand. The body remains faced to the side and the feeling is of strong contraction.

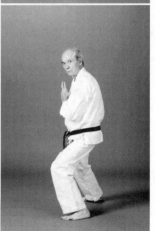

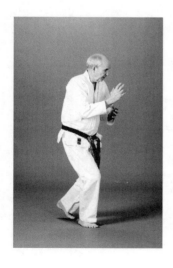

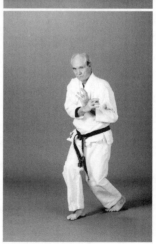

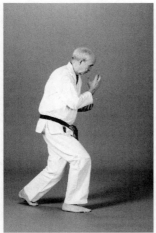

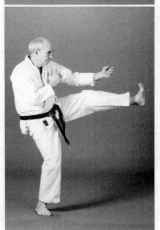

19. Seamlessly rebound off the contraction with a strong expansion into a left front stamping kick at diaphragm level and a simultaneous left-hand upper level thrust with the phantom ball, which has transferred from the right hand at the beginning of the expansion.

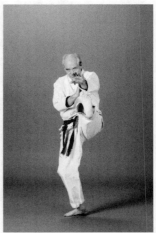

20. Step strongly down to the front with the left foot while retracting back and transferring the phantom ball to the right hand. Continue seamlessly on into a step forward with the right leg while thrusting to the upper level with the phantom ball.

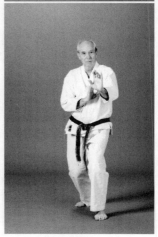

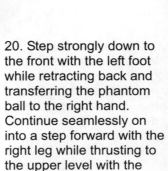

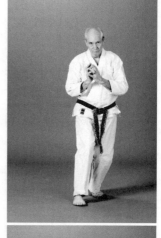

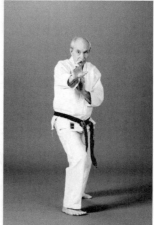

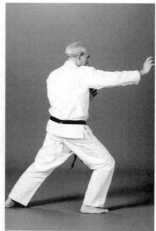

21. Pivot to the rear in place, contracting strongly down into a sweeping right-hand middle level forearm block while coiling down and in. The left hand comes around to the guard position as shown. The body is inclined somewhat to the front and the weight is largely on the rear leg.

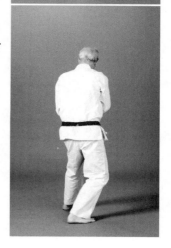

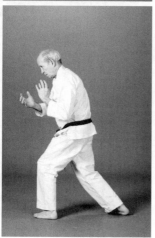

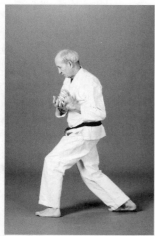

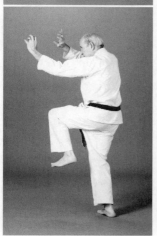

22. Seamlessly rebound off the contraction, uncoiling expansively up into a "thunder step" (stamp) with the right leg while executing a thrusting block up and in with both arms to unbalance the opponent. The phantom ball transfers to the left hand just at the beginning of the movement. The left leg comes up dynamically with the body. The left foot is at the inside of the right knee.

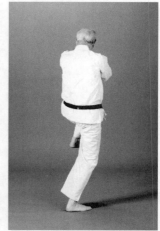

23. Step strongly down and to the front with the left leg while retracting back and transferring the phantom ball to the right hand. Continue seamlessly on into a step forward with the right leg while executing an upper level thrust with the phantom ball.

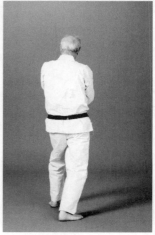

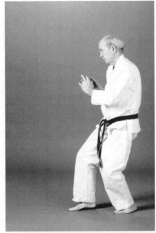

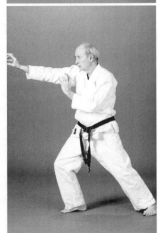

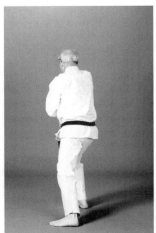

Return to the upright combat posture.

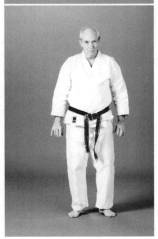

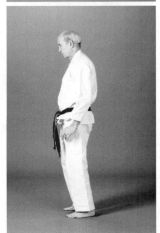

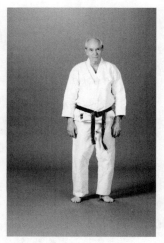

Assume a natural stance.

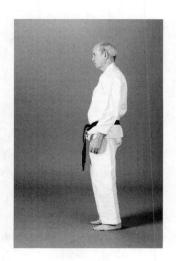

## Balancing the Phantom Ball Form

Repeat the above ball form balancing process with the phantom ball. Balancing this form in its slower format can give some really good insight on your basic all-round mobility.

L7. Stand up on the left leg. The right foot rests at the inside of the left knee. Look to the right. The right hand is in a guard position in front of the sternum or makes a down block. The phantom ball is held overhead in the left hand.

L8. Step down to the right with the right leg, simultaneously sweeping down and out to the front with both hands and just slightly across to the right. The hands retract and the phantom ball shifts to the right hand.

L9-L10. Flow into an expansion striking out to the upper level with the phantom ball in the right hand while simultaneously executing an upper level block with the left arm.

L11-L12. Both hands pull strongly back with the body turning strongly to the left while the left leg simultaneously steps forward across the right leg. The right hand with the phantom ball sweeps across to the left at shoulder level while the left hand sweeps down across at knee level.

L13. Stand up strongly on the left leg, the body uncoiling to the front. At the beginning of this movement the phantom ball transfers to the left hand, which thrusts the phantom ball forward at face level. The right hand comes to the guard position or pulling hand. The right leg comes up dynamically with the strong left hip movement. The right foot is at the inside left knee level.

Look to the right and raise the phantom ball overhead. Repeat L7 through L13 until it feels natural and then move to the next set of techniques.

L16. Stand in the position at the end of move 16 with the right foot forward and the left foot back. The phantom ball is in the right hand.

L17. Step in deeply with the left leg. At the beginning of the step the phantom ball transfers to the left hand and then strikes at the tantien level. The right hand is in the guard position in front of the chest.

L18. Look to the rear and step back and behind the left leg with the right leg. At the same time the left hand sweeps the phantom ball across the body at face level from left to right. The right hand moves with the left hand. The body remains faced to the side and the feeling is of strong contraction.

L19. Quickly rebound off the contraction with strong expansion into a right front stamping kick at diaphragm level and a simultaneous right-hand upper level thrust with the phantom ball, which has transferred from the left hand at the beginning of the expansion.

L20. Step strongly down to the front with the right foot while retracting back and transferring the phantom ball to the left hand. Continue seamlessly on into a step forward with the left leg while thrusting to the upper level with the phantom ball.

You are now in the approximate position of the end of L16. Look to the rear and repeat L16 through L20 until they feel natural then move to the final set of techniques.

L21. Stand in the final position of L20. Then pivot to the rear in place contracting strongly down into a sweeping left-hand forearm block while coiling down and in. The right hand comes around to the guard position. The body inclines somewhat to the front and the weight is largely on the rear leg.

L22. Quickly rebound off the contraction, uncoiling expansively up into a "thunder step" (stamp) with the left leg while executing a thrusting block in and up with both arms to unbalance the opponent. The phantom ball is transferred to the right hand just at the beginning of the movement. The right leg comes up dynamically with the body. The right foot is at the left knee.

L23. Step strongly down and to the front with the right leg retracting back and transferring the phantom ball to the left hand. Continue seamlessly on into a step forward with the left leg while executing an upper level thrust with the phantom ball.

Repeat L21 through L23 until they feel natural. Then add in the simpler parts to the form and do the form from the beginning. After some repetition the whole form will feel natural.

## Empty Hands Form

Unlike the ball and staff versions, the empty hands version allows full and free use of both hands. The alternative hand positions in moves 8, 13, 17, and 18 were influenced by the differing nuances of the ball and the staff. The original hand version was influenced by the staff. Without the ball in mind, the pulling/withdrawing movements can be made larger for a more dynamic feel as contrasted with the more combat-oriented guard position. At the time I felt this was great for the empty arm concept. I currently use both guard and full pulling/withdrawing movements about equally for this form. This is because my withdrawing side and empty arm understanding has improved. The contrast between the two hand positions has been instructional.

The ball was less familiar at the beginning and I was slower to apply it to changes in my technique. As I worked more with the ball, I ended up with two empty hand versions (phantom ball and empty hands) for contrast in order to shed light on internalizing and empty arm technique.

It is clear to me that internalizing and the empty arm concepts are inseparable — not two sides of the same coin, more like two of the sides of a die.

The foot positions for each of the moves are shown in the ball form.

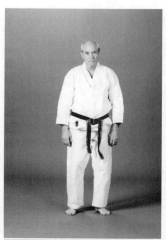

Stand naturally.

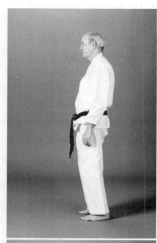

1. Assume the combat posture. Awareness extends in all directions. See, feel, and hear the room. Stand with the arms at the sides, both palms facing the floor.

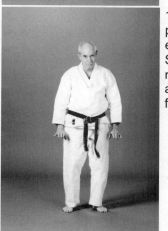

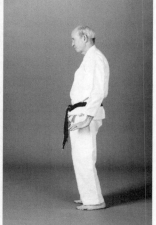

2. Step forward into a ready position, left foot forward. Both hands come up into a guard position. They may be open or clenched. Weight is about 70% on the rear leg.

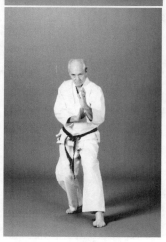

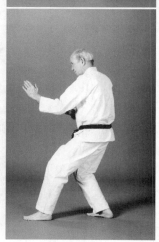

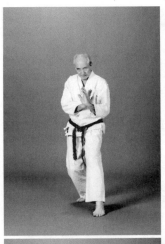

3. Take a short sliding step forward with the left leg.

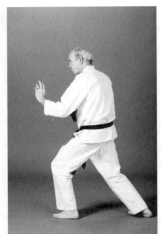

4. Take a full step forward with the right leg.

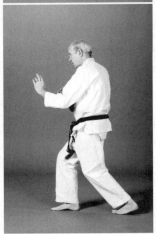

5. Take a full step forward with the left leg. During these first movements the feeling is of awareness in all directions while smoothly and carefully walking forward.

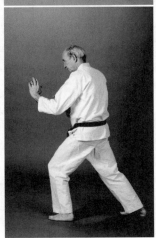

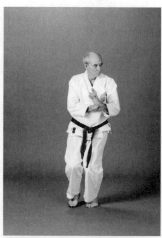

6. Step forward with the right leg simultaneously looking to the left. Shift your awareness more strongly, but not completely, to the left where the most threatening opponent is. Until the end of the form, awareness rests primarily but not completely in the direction of the major threat. Critical edge orientation follows awareness.

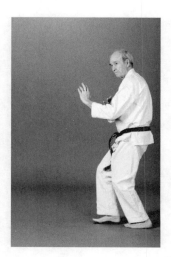

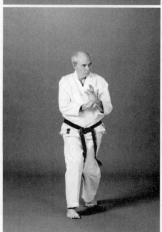

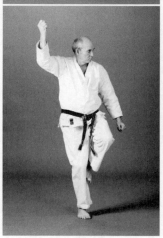

7. Stand up on the right leg with a strong expansive feeling. The left foot rises dynamically to the inside of the right knee. The right hand rises up just above the head and the left hand sweeps down to the left side.

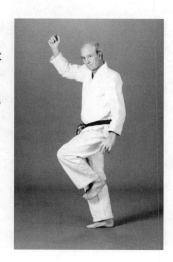

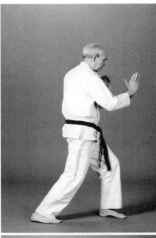

8. Step down to the left with the left leg simultaneously sweeping down across and to the front with the right hand to execute a middle level block. The left hand comes up to a middle level guard position or it may come around to the traditional hip "pulling hand" position for a more dynamic feel. The feeling is that of a large spring-like contraction after the large expansion of the previous move. The weight is just slightly more to the front.

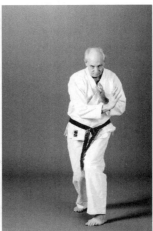

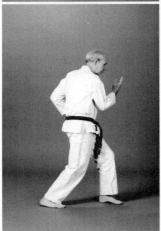

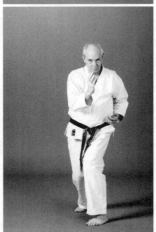

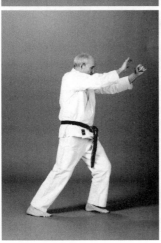

9-11. Immediately rebound off the contraction with a simultaneous left-hand, close-range upper level attack and a right-hand upper level block/ disruption. There is some feeling of expansion and of getting in with a small weight shift forward at the end of the hand movements. The hands recoil back into a guard position.

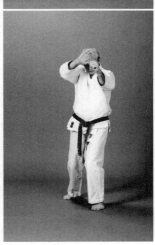

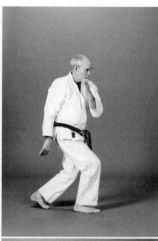

12. Seamlessly step forward across the left leg with the right leg as shown while strongly turning the body to the right, simultaneously sweeping down across the body to the right lower level with the right hand and across to the middle level with the left hand. The feeling is of an inwardly coiling contraction.

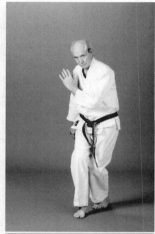

13. Stand up strongly on the right leg, the body uncoiling to the front with a strong feeling of expansion. The right hand simultaneously thrusts forward in an upper level attack. The left hand comes to the left hip pulling hand position (or a guard position to more closely match the staff form). The left leg comes up dynamically with the strong right hip movement as shown.

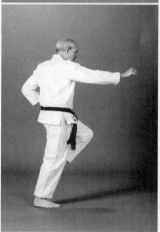

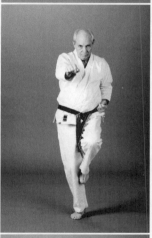

14. Instantly step down and strongly forward a half step with the left leg. Awareness shifts more strongly to the rear. The left hand can be in a guard position or used as a pulling hand.

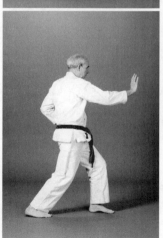

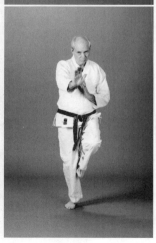

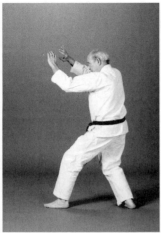

15. Quickly step forward with the right leg while turning to the rear and execute upper level blocks with both arms as shown. The weight is more on the right leg.

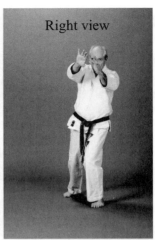

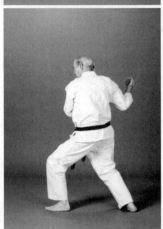

16. Sweep both arms back to the middle level as shown with a feeling of getting in and a slight weight shift forward.

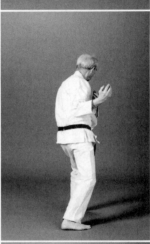

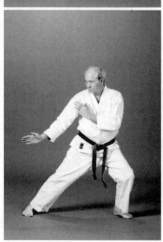

17. Step in deeply and expansively with the right leg while thrusting to the tantien level with the right hand. The left hand is in the guard position or the left hip. If this were not following the movements of the staff form, the strike might be transferred to middle level. Steps 15, 16, and 17 are executed as one seamless unit.

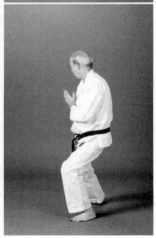

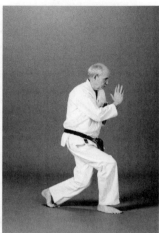

18. Look to the rear and step back, across, and behind the right leg with the left leg. At the same time the right hand sweeps across the body from right to left in an upper level block and the left comes to a middle level guard position or to the left hip. The body remains faced to the side and the feeling is of strong contraction.

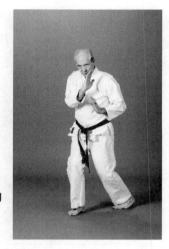

19. Seamlessly rebound off the contraction with a strong expansion into a diaphragm level left front stamping kick and a simultaneous upper level, left-hand eye attack.

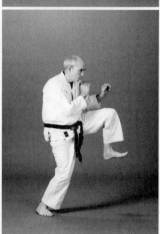

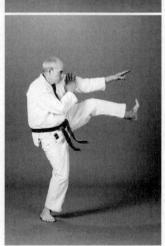

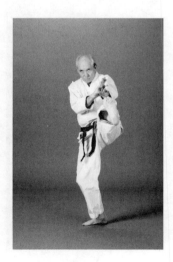

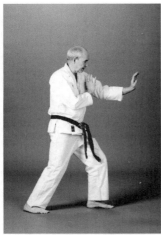

20. Step strongly down to the front with the left leg and then continue on into a step forward with the right leg while executing a right-hand upper level punch.

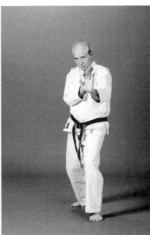

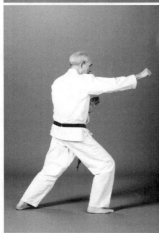

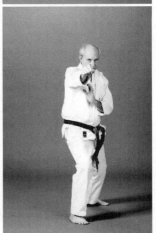

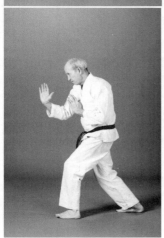

21. Pivot to the rear in place, contracting strongly into an upper level right-hand block coming across and in from right to left. The body has coiled down and in. The left hand comes to a middle level guard position or to the left hip. The body inclines somewhat to the front and the weight is a bit more on the rear leg.

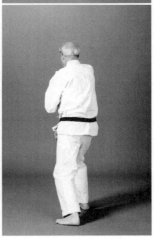

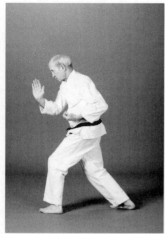

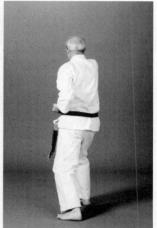

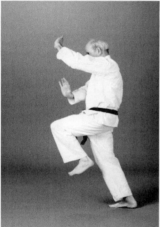

22. Rebound seamlessly off the contraction, uncoiling up expansively into a "thunder step" (stamp) while executing double-arm thrusting blocks as shown in and up to unbalance the opponent. The left leg comes up dynamically and stops with the foot at the right knee.

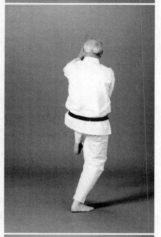

23. Step strongly down and to the front with the left leg and then continue on into a step forward with the right leg while executing an upper level right-hand punch.

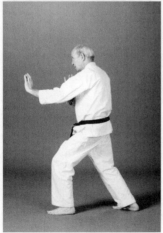

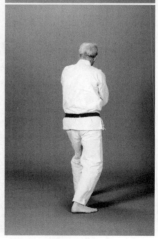

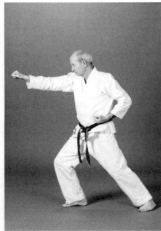

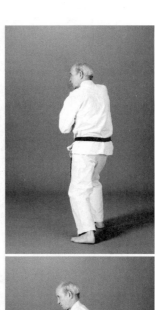

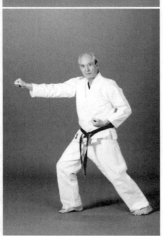

Return to the upright combat position.

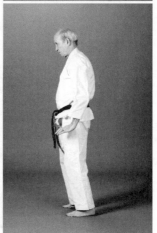

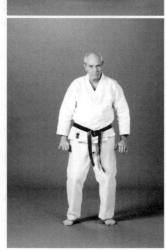

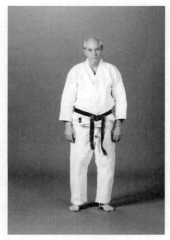

Assume a natural posture.

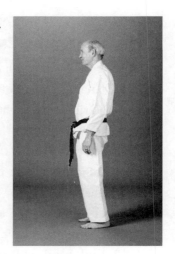

## Balancing the Empty Hands Form

Balancing the empty hands form is similar to balancing in the other forms.

L7. Stand up on the left leg. The right foot rests at the inside of the left knee. Look to the right. The right hand makes a down block. The left hand rises to just above the head.

L8. Step down to the right with the right leg, simultaneously sweeping down and out to the front with the left hand in a middle level block. The right hand goes to a guard position or the right hip.

L9-L11. Flow into an expansion striking out to the upper level with the right hand while simultaneously executing an upper level block with the left arm.

L12. Both hands pull strongly back with the body turning strongly to the left while the left leg simultaneously steps forward across the right leg. The right hand sweeps across to the left at shoulder level while the left hand sweeps down across at knee level.

L13. Stand up strongly on the left leg, the body uncoiling to the front. Punch with the left hand at face level. The right hand comes to the guard position or pulling hand. The right leg comes up dynamically with the strong left hip movement. The right foot is at the inside left knee level.

Look to the right and raise the phantom ball overhead. Repeat L7 through L13 until it feels natural and then move to the next set of techniques.

L16. Stand in the position at the end of move 16 with the right foot forward and the left foot back.

L17. Step in deeply with the left leg. The left hand strikes at the tantien level. The right hand is in the guard position in front of the chest or on the right hip.

L18. Look to the rear and step back and behind the left leg with the right leg. At the same time the left hand sweeps across the body at face level from left to right. The right hand goes to a guard position. The body remains faced to the side and the feeling is of strong contraction.

L19. Quickly rebound off the contraction with strong expansion into a right front stamping kick at diaphragm level and a simultaneous right-hand eye attack.

L20. Step strongly down to the front with the right foot. Continue seamlessly on into a step forward with the left leg while executing a left-hand upper level punch.

You are now in the approximate position of the end of L16. Look to the rear and repeat L16 through L20 until they feel natural then move to the final set of techniques.

L21. Stand in the final position of L20. Then pivot to the rear in place contracting strongly down into a sweeping left-hand forearm block while coiling down and in. The right hand comes around to the guard position. The body inclines somewhat to the front and the weight is largely on the rear leg.

L22. Quickly rebound off the contraction, uncoiling expansively up into a "thunder step" (stamp) with the left leg while executing a thrusting block in and up with both arms to unbalance the opponent. The right leg comes up dynamically with the body. The right foot is at the left knee.

L23. Step strongly down and to the front with the right leg. Continue seamlessly on into a step forward with the left leg while executing an upper level left-hand punch.

Repeat L21 through L23 until they feel natural. Then add in the simpler parts to the form and do the form from the beginning. After some repetition the whole form will feel natural.

# 5. Sparring and Mobility Drills

Ideal mobility would be effectively moving against opponents in accordance with all the principles and concepts. Ideal mobility is probably beyond the reach of most but there is no excuse for not trying. Movement drills are invaluable in developing effective, practical mobility. They can be done without opponents (shadow boxing) or with opponents. There are also excellent drills with equipment, either used by oneself or handled by training partners. A few of these are described below.

The various arts have a huge number of drills. Introduction or adaptation of the ball into some of the many drills and exercises can be quite valuable. As mentioned before, boxers such as Lamon Brewster and my training partners, the Shaver brothers, get good results with ball work adaptations to their drills. A fellow karate practitioner has adapted the ball to his study of the yoga chakras and is very enthusiastic regarding the results. He reported a significant increase in the energizing effect of several exercises.

# Basic Ball Management/Maneuver Drills

## Step One: Moving around without an Opponent

Use your lightest ball to begin with. Hold the ball as shown in the preliminary exercises. This is a basic combat hand position and makes these drills a natural/logical extension of the preliminary exercises.

The tactile hands and feet integrate and act simultaneously with the center/centers. Move around feeling that the hands, feet, and center are moving in an integrated whole-body manner.

Shadow box, use your favorite offensive techniques and defensive maneuvers.

Note that mentally lingering over a move or a mistake really interrupts the flow when maneuvering with a ball. This is a real virtue of ball practice. You soon find that you need to be mentally just ahead of the ball and stay there. Intent, opponent connection, room awareness, and self-assessment occur at the same time. Obviously this mental and physical multi-tasking is important in combat and requires close attention. The drills below are a basic introduction to multi-tasking with the ball, which then morphs into staff and equipment drills.

## Step Two: Movement with an Opponent

Before exposing your friend to your ball expertise, you should warm up and get "calibrated" with your ball.

Important safety point, you and your opponent should be wearing shoes. Start with your lightest ball.

### Following

Have an opponent assume a somewhat long combat distance and maneuver evasively. The opponent should start at a very moderate pace. Follow the opponent maintaining the long combat distance while the hands stay on the combat line. The hands steer the ball to follow the opponent in coordination with the action of the feet and center/centers in maintaining the basic combat line directly to the opponent. As following your opponent's evasions becomes familiar, try to feel that the hands (especially the fingers), the center, and the feet (especially the toes) are acting simultaneously.

By combat line, I mean that the ideal combat line for you is one where you have all your best weapons aligned and available against your opponent and you are behind him or have otherwise positioned yourself to negate his preferred weapons. For this basic exercise the combat line has the opponent pretty much directly in front of you but with some advantageous angle adjustments.

For these exercises, initially concentrate on maintaining your maximum offensive capability while maneuvering. Do not be fixated on offense, but always maintain the capability. Do not be concerned with your partners' weapons; just follow his changes as instantaneously and smoothly as you can. Gradually focus on strategic combined offensive/defensive maneuvering like Jack Dempsey, as discussed below on page 220.

### Evading

Next have the opponent move aggressively towards you while you maneuver evasively, maintaining the hands and center/centers on the combat line. Try to feel that the hands, centers, and feet act simultaneously, as above, in maneuvering. As you become more adept, try to time the evasions closer to the opponent's full commitment to his move and also gain a superior combat position. Gradually focus on Dempsey-like, combined offensive/defensive techniques.

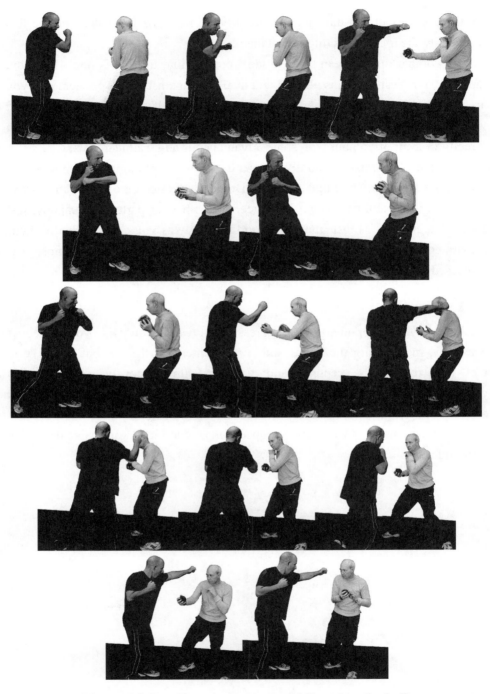

**Figure 76: Evading an opponent while using the ball.**

### Following and Evading on the Critical Edge

When the two drills above are familiar and you and your opponent seem to be pretty well coordinated with a smooth flow, work the drills while on the critical edge. Feel that with the slightest extra mental or physical effort you could instantly thrust the ball into the opponent and that while maneuvering forward, backward, or to the side the thrusts would have effective force.

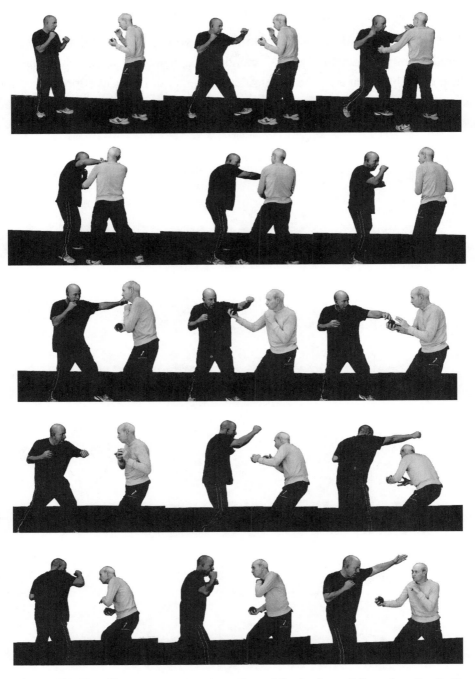

**Figure 77: Evading an opponent on the critical edge while using the ball.**

### Ball Attacks Following and Evading

Next open the distance up a just bit, just out of contact range for your partner's safety.

Thrust at the opponent with the ball. Follow the opponent as before when he moves evasively. Begin with a very measured pace. Try to stay on the critical edge as you follow his evasions with your attacks. Your feet, centers, and hands should move together as you herd the opponent around.

Assume the evasive role. While the opponent tries to herd you, maneuver on the critical edge and maintain a series of accurate, timely attacks to the opponent.

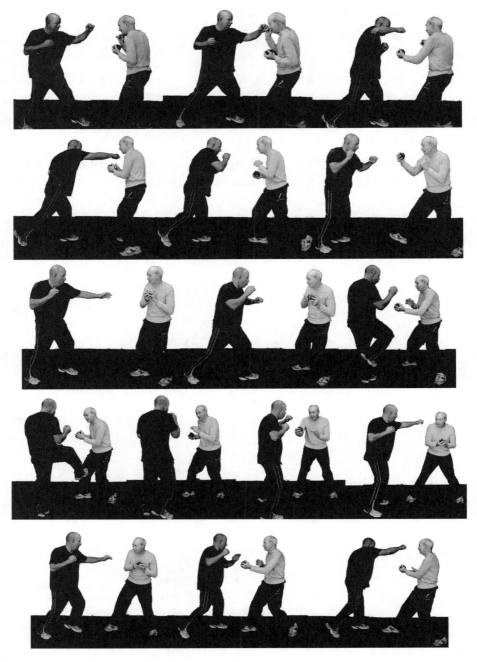

**Figure 78: Maneuver and thrust with ball at opponent while he evades and/or counters, both on the critical edge and just outside of contact range.**

**Combat Distance Ball Attacks, Following, Evading**

When you and your opponent are in sync, begin working in to real combat distance and maintain the effectiveness of your attacks. This is not easy to do. Archie Moore said that he knew Mohammed Ali was the real deal when he saw him punch effectively while moving backwards.

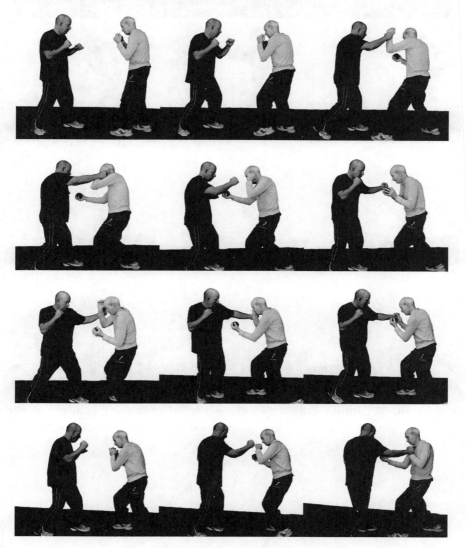

**Figure 79: On the critical edge attack and follow the opponent using the ball to maneuver and strike.**

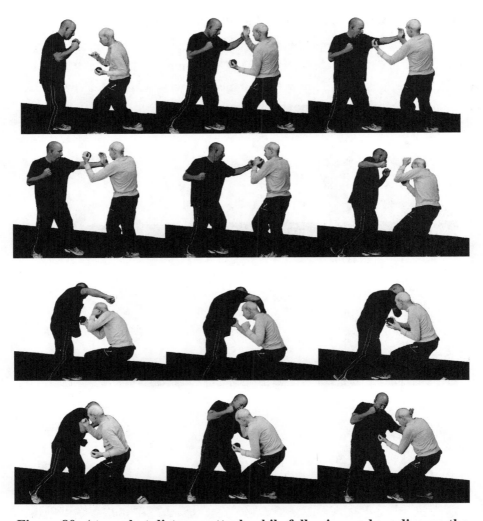

**Figure 80: At combat distance attack while following and evading on the critical edge.**

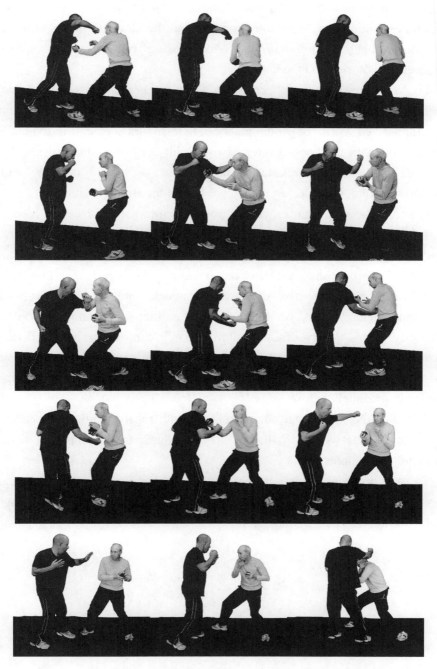

**Figure 81: At combat distance, on critical edge, follow, evade, attack.**

While doing all this, keep your awareness of the room, a good flow, etc. Sometimes focus strongly on the opponent and the strategic battle. Other times focus on what is happening with your body in using your hands, centers, and feet to maneuver yourself and the ball.

Lu Wen Wei's multiple centers concept integrated with flow, breathing (abdominal and reverse abdominal), while on the critical edge should be one of the emphasized parts of your practice here. Work centers individually in combination with the upper center, always with the knees and with the fingers and toes as movement initiators. The objective is instant mobility with an appropriate strike, block, or evasion according to the strategic situation.

Practicing this with an especially good training partner recently brought an appreciation of the mobility nuances of the upper two centers. I felt like I was fighting a ghost. In *Spalding's Book on Boxing and Physical Culture* by Thomas Inch, James Corbett observed that contrary to popular belief, Jack Dempsey did not bob and weave defensively. Instead his attacks included defensively viable body movement. This is what my training partner was doing so effectively. Obviously this is a very desirable ability and it can also be reversed to good effect by including well-timed strikes or disruptive contacts within an evasion practice. You can test your striking effectiveness for this in the equipment practice immediately below.

IMPORTANT: Use your common sense with regards to the pace when you are in close range with the ball. Do not force the speed beyond your ability to safeguard your opponent.

To develop an appreciation of the withdrawing side in mobility, repeat the exercises above with the ball held as much as possible in the withdrawing side hand. (See internalizing on page 230.)

## *Ball Combat Drills*

These drills are somewhat more reality-based than the above introductory drills.

After developing good expertise in the above drills, concentrate on maneuver that denies your partners their weapons and/or preferred combat style. Needless to say, partners with a variety of combat styles are highly desirable. Their versatility will challenge your ball handling and maneuvering abilities and enhance your skills.

Modify your own art's combat drills to safely use the ball with them in order to study any of the above ideas and concepts that interest you. It certainly does not have to be your own art; the many excellent combat drills of the various martial arts are a fertile ground for adaptation and study.

When you are moving well and are tuned in to the maneuvering, lose the opponent and shadow box with the ball. You can visualize an opponent or work on any aspect of the ball practice you wish. Try your personal combat style with the ball. Visualize a known opponent, someone who presents a real problem. Personally I do a lot of specific opponent visualization in all areas of my practice and find it very rewarding. I think that most would agree that there are those "nightmare" opponents where it's not a question of being competitive, but where the issue is survival. These opponents really make you focus and think about all aspects of your practice.

### Reality Gaps

An observation frequently made is that many advanced combat drills labor under the "illusion of control." That is to say there is a conscious or unconscious assumption that it is usually probable that one can dictate the distance, timing, or even the form of a real fight.

Since training usually occurs within a relatively closed group, it is easy to become comfortable and relatively unquestioning about one's practice.

I well recall the shock of many when the striking arts fighters encountered the grapplers in the full contact bouts held relatively recently. Actually this is not a new phenomenon. Grapplers have always been the bane of pure strikers, especially in the more limiting, sporting-type matches.

Internalizing ability can bring some balance to the situation. Effectively striking from even a beaten posture is possible and should be a major goal. I believe that the ball practice can be quite helpful for this.

For the striking arts, finding grapplers to mutually explore martial arts with would be good. Some of this already occurs. Add some weapons people into the mix and epiphanies will abound. The Dog Brothers have had a version of this for years. Check out their videos.

Those so inclined could work on the "dark side," using offensive/defensive techniques like knee breaking or eye attacks, which are foolishly ignored by many. Most martial arts styles do have these realistic techniques, but many seem to put them on the back burner or just give them lip service.

## *Staff Maneuvering Practice*

Repeat the ball maneuvering format with the staff. This is an excellent practice because you can use hard contact techniques if you have the equipment mentioned below. Start with rather light contact and increase the intensity as familiarity develops.

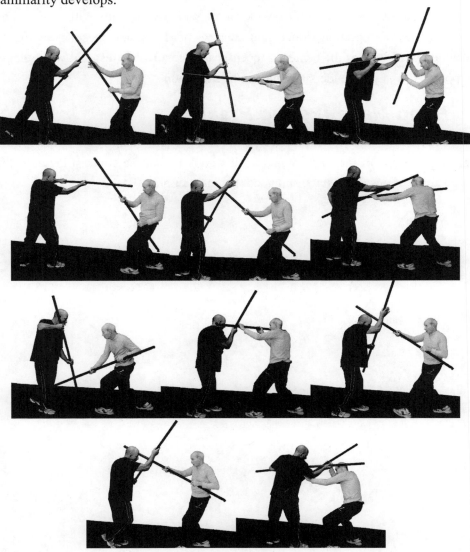

**Figure 82: Maneuvering with staffs. Note occasional light contact.**

Note how critical edge maintenance enhances your flow and remember to pay attention to the role of the withdrawing side and cross loading in technique execution.

Be sure to explore Lu Wen Wei's middle center concept; the virtue of the multi-vector rotating ball visualization becomes obvious. Work it with the upper center, then try the three-centers model as a whole.

Also be especially certain to work on the withdrawing side with mother line and centering integration. Since you can use hard contact, these internalizing techniques, as well as the centers concept, can face a reality test that will quickly expose flaws in your understanding and/or execution.

## *Hand Maneuvering Practice*

Repeat the maneuver practice with your regular hand and foot striking techniques. One of the main points of this book is that the contrast between the three applications (ball, staff, and hands) is instructional.

## *Advanced Drills*

Try the basic ball management and maneuver drills with the ball held as much as possible on the withdrawing side.

Repeat the ball thrusting part of the earlier drills with your fists and maneuver using striking mitts and body armor or fight shields. This can be very productive since you are really striking and can get feedback on your progress.

As you get really tuned in to it the "opponent" can occasionally jam or evade and test your rebound management. With the mitts and body armor, the opponent can also add occasional counters after your strikes or after disrupting you. This will test your awareness/transitions/flow sense and also give you practical centering experience.

### Withdrawing Side

There are some specific withdrawing side bag drills that help you "taste" the concept. Here are a couple of them.

With an Escrima stick held in one hand, strike the bag as shown on page 105. Note the effectiveness of your strikes.

Now hold the stick with the other hand placed on the stick hand wrist as shown on page 106. Strike the bag in the same pattern as before with power emphasis on the withdrawing side. Note how the palms basically tend to face each other as in the ball handling. Most note a considerable power increase with the hands united.

Now go beyond the basic practice by integrating the middle center action with the toes, fingers, and lower center all working the stick. Focus is on withdrawing side awareness, but be aware of the mother line and its extensions, which are significant here for maintaining balanced structure.

Add body shifting, flowing into seamless vector changes with a whole-body character.

Maneuver on the bag, striking in from many angles as you might in a fight. Then separate the hands just a bit, but accompany the stick hand with the augmenting hand and with the palms facing each other. Use the separated hand side with the same emphasis as when the hands were united. Your goal is to generate force somewhat equal to the united hand practice. Next use a light ball in the augmenting hand. This is very good for internalizing. Note that if you concentrate on maneuvering the ball and relaxing the stick side around the mother line axis, the amount of force is enhanced.

Strike a bag with a staff using the same basic format as with the stick. The front hand is the targeting hand. The rear hand is the power hand.

## Rebound

One of the best descriptions of how to work with rebound comes from a post by Joel Weinberg on one of his web forums. I have cut and cropped this post to focus on it as an example of a good way to take a common practice (in this case, hitting a heavy bag) and configure it to study an important concept, such as rebound. This type of deconstructive process leads to deeper levels of understanding, or at least deeper levels of questions. The drill offers very good insight on some important aspects of internalizing. Here is what Joel had to say:

> Rebound: to bounce back. In terms of our martial arts, the energy which we attempt to impart to the target can, if not managed, bounce back or be absorbed by our own body, dissipating its energy transmission to the target.

> Example — Like a stick you swing and hit a brick wall with, the vibration coming back up the stick to your hand is rebound. That is, the energy is returning back through the stick to the hand holding it.

> In terms of rebound, we have to examine how it is created in the body and why it occurs.

> A linear punch, structurally supported, still will receive rebound if the muscles are not properly engaged or disengaged. This is also true with the rotational punch.

> A linear punch is supported by an aligned, interconnected structure. A rotational punch ALSO HAS INTERCONNECTED STRUCTURE! The difference in the latter is that the power generated does not primarily rely on structural (skeletal) support, but internally the SAME PRINCIPLES MUST APPLY, as the

internal structure STILL MUST WORK TOGETHER AS ONE BODY UNIT. The WHOLE of the body must be behind the strike, either rotational or linear; all must be interconnected to work properly.

Examples of why rebound occurs in either punch:

Tension in the body. At the point of tension, or rigidity, the body will lose the internal connectedness, reducing forward energy transfer.

Localization of strength (similar to above). When impact occurs, the energy must go somewhere. If, for example, the shoulder is tight or poorly aligned, energy from the impact is looking for a weak link, so to speak. The shoulder muscle loads, and resistance is localized there. The force is taken into the shoulder, and the unitized connection broken. If misaligned, the force diverts from the target. This can occur with either rotational or straight punching.

Prolonged contact with the target. Especially when striking with a rotational punch, at impact there must be an immediate transfer of energy to the target. This is critical to understand. One MUST RELEASE THE PUNCH. To not release the punch, the energy will dissipate back into one's own body. In terms of the linear punch, there is the kinetic impact of travel and momentum, and the body unit itself is structurally driving in and supporting the punch. But, if the arm is too tight, or the chest is engaged, the chain once again is broken and the punch will take rebound.

This is a bit difficult to get if one is not used to using aligned structure. But even at impact, the body is very much disengaged with regard to muscle tension. This goes back to structural (skeletal) support of the aligned punch. So, if one makes an attempt to forcefully drive in the punch and tension occurs, the chain of connection of the linear punch will be broken at the point of tension and will take rebound.

With regard to changing fist angles, inclusive of rotation of the body, the arm being bent, at odd angles, etc, what is important is what occurs at impact. We must remember that weight in motion with speed makes for good impact. So we come back to developing interconnected structure in rotation. Either linear or rotational, certain principles must be trained in the body.

As a small example, consider an eight-pound shot-putt suspended by a cord. Swing it around and hit someone with it. It could easily kill, yet there is no linear connection to the ground to support it. Consider that you could do the same by transferring your weight through core rotation out to your hand or fist, with no tension inhibiting its impact. It's a good idea but this is not so easy, how DO we transfer the energy and eliminate the undue tension that creates rebound?

To feel what we are describing, try this.

I suggest that you proceed carefully with this. The most difficult aspect of this is to KNOW WHAT TO FEEL. You have to know the different nuances to clearly read your rebound. I state again, once you learn how to feel what needs to be released, you will become much of your own teacher.

Use a heavy bag for this drill. Heavy enough to offer fair resistance, light enough to move.

Practice good rotational crosses in the air, back foot pivoting on the ball of the foot.

Go to the bag, throw the cross with moderate force; and at impact, strive to drive it on in. What you will feel in your arm/shoulder is rebound. While doing it again, engage or raise your chest. You will feel a different rebound.

Next, DON'T hit the bag yet, get loose, easy. Throw loosely, easily, relaxed punches in the air. Get the feel of the body all moving together. CRITICAL — feel your chest relax, drop out of the way, and be aware of your back, your hip, legs... and get the feel of your body sort of dropping into the punch/bag.

Now on the bag, don't try to hit hard, but gradually increase the velocity of the strike, and all together throw, rotate, and feel as if you allow the hand to drop in, penetrate, and release at impact. Important — be aware of your back, slightly snug. This is hard to explain in writing, but allow the chest to relax, and the back to be doing much of the work. Increase speed, and time your impact and release. The whole body moves together; easy pivot on the ball of the back foot, body drops in, no tension in arm, arm connected to back, chest disengaged, and shoulder NOT forcing the punch.

Not forcing the punch does not mean that it is not explosive or is low impact. It means to allow the impact by full body mechanics, the feel and the energy focus to be as one. The end result is explosive with full unity and no push, seamlessly releasing after impact.

Go back to trying to "punch hard," and see the difference.

Always remember to NOT force the punch and to release at the end. Once contact is made, ideally the energy is transferred to the target. You are done and seamlessly into the next technique. Remember to release. You are not hitting with the hand/arm. You are hitting with the core energy of the body being transferred out through the hand/fist.

This bag drill touches on important points such as no local tension, "lingering" is bad, seamless flowing into the next movement is good, whole-body movement, core energy transfer, withdrawing side understanding, and, of course, rebound management.

I have some suggestions for using and enhancing the valuable understanding offered here, and for attacking the questions you may have about the process.

Work through it until you get the points Joel is making. Then hold a light ball in the non-striking hand and work the bag with rebound in mind. This is good for studying how to internalize empty arm, withdrawing side/core energy transference and provides a different "look" at your rebound management.

Maneuver on the bag as you would normally while doing bag work, taking no rebound except that which aids maneuver. Try to maximize transference of core energy to the striking hand without interrupting breathing and flow and be sure to maintain the critical edge. Try your best and worst combinations until each punch manages rebound fairly well and you are consistently transferring core energy with both hands to some extent. Remember, intelligently designed combinations end with defensive moves: bobbing, weaving, warding, jabbing, etc.

Finally, when you have confidence in your understanding and application, "fight" the bag. As the bag swings around, visualize it striking at you, evade and counter, occasionally striking or warding off from awkward positions while managing rebound and generating good core energy transference.

Take the understanding gained from this drill and apply it to the internalizing, withdrawing side, and other drills we have already looked at.

Bag work is a truly productive training method. Personally I might even call it a Big Deal. The above bag exercise illustrates its value.

## Internalizing

The maneuver practices above and the staff sparring practice below, once very familiar to you, are good places to explore and test internalizing your technique.

You have heard of things being two sides of the same coin. Well internalizing with its withdrawing side, core energy transference, empty arm, rebound management, structural integration, and whole-body applications are all different sides of the same die (dice). The various elements should be considered as leading to a multi-faceted whole.

Some sides of the die will be more of a problem than others. Feedback from your training partners is an essential factor in solving the problems. For example, there is a tendency in sparring to focus more on the mobility and timing techniques of successful offensive and defensive maneuver than on the nuts and bolts of effective structural maneuver; this is a mistake. Effective structure results in effective technique. Application of an ineffective technique at the end of a successful maneuver is definitely not the goal here. Your training partners can feel your relative internalizing lethality more certainly than you can estimate it. Awareness of the varying training goals of individuals is important for progress of the group as a whole. Internalizing is nuanced, quite subtle, as progress is made. As stated before, it is a "gateway" concept that leads to other significant questions; it deserves considerable attention. All training partners should be on the same page in this. Noting increased power with less motion in the equipment drills and the rebound drill above would be an example. Also, training partners can note other important considerations, such as breath regulation, which is critical to successful internalizing. Internalizing is improving when effective power is generated while the withdrawing side hand remains in the indisputably useful guard position. Training partners can test this point until the guard is reflexive.

## Balancing Combat Drills

In most martial arts there are combat drills that focus on particular aspects of the overall combat method. I feel that the drills should be balanced right/left side and also include techniques for getting to the preferred side or to the opponent's weak side (if he has one). This is the same concept as the grappling arts getting opponents to their domain, the ground.

# Staff Sparring

I feel that sparring with the safer flexible type of weapons and protective gear cited below has exceptional merit and that this is true on many levels. This is one of the few practices that offers a venue to realistically "taste" and test understanding of flow, maneuver, centers, withdrawing side, internalizing, etc.

The equipment, while not universally available, is fairly accessible. This about as close to real combat as relative beginners can experience in order to safely guide their practice. It is important for students to have a clear vision of "real" combat for setting their martial arts goals early on in their training rather than relying on mere words or just observation.

As one progresses, this practice provides practical insight into your combat strengths and weaknesses.

There is a lot of the safer weaponry available besides the staff. If you have the protective equipment and willing training partners you can experience some really insightful and versatile practice.

## Staff Sparring Equipment

For practicing forms use the size and type of staff you favor. For sparring, the ones made from white polyvinyl chloride (PVC) plastic plumbing pipe with a rubber shell have some real advantages. The shock absorbing flexibility of this staff allows you to really swat your opponent without any significant damage. This has the advantage of realistic attacking biomechanics. Matches where attacks are pulled have a built in balancing mechanism that would not be present in real combat where you are attacking into or through your opponent. If you are really trying to attack your opponent and you miss or your opponent skillfully deflects you, you can have a real problem. You might even say you can have a reality problem. Harold Gunns, a very fine boxing coach, taught us that first you learn how to hit, and then you learn how to miss. Real contact sparring is reality sparring. The main problem with real contact is that there is some difficulty in conserving brain cells and other important body parts. Relatively safe staffs and a bit of protective gear are a reasonable compromise.

The PVC staffs do have one drawback. They are much more flexible than wooden staffs. They can flex quite a bit during swinging strikes and make contact, whereas a wooden staff would be stopped. This is unrealistic in terms of your blocking ability. A real fighting staff would not flex that much, so your defensive sense could be misinformed. Of course there are some Chinese bai-la (wax wood) staffs that are designed to be quite flexible, probably to flex around your block and whack your head.

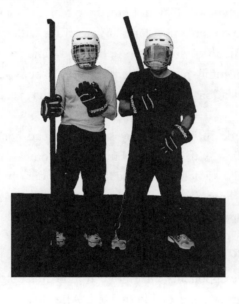

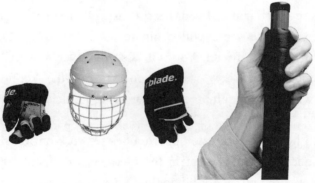

**Figure 83: Protective gear for realistic sparring.**

Street hockey gloves, headgear with face shields, safety goggles, kneepads, and elbow pads are usually enough for most people. Shoes are also useful because foot attacks are a very good sneak attack and feet are quite vulnerable to thrusts from the ends of the staff.

## Individual Bouts

Staff bouts should begin with individual sparring. If you are used to weapons sparring, you already know that an immediate benefit is a new dimension to your distance sense. If you have not done any sparring with weapons, you may find that it is more difficult to soften the upper body and to control your breathing. Your stamina is definitely more challenged. Whole-body technique with effective mother line application really helps the stamina issue, as does breathing understanding.

Be sure to work on balancing by switching lead hands and lead legs. This seems strange at first with weapons but soon becomes functional. Work for the ability to smoothly switch back and forth without giving openings to your opponents. Notice how switching lead hands gives you new angles to maneuver and attack your opponents.

## Multiple Opponent Bouts

Start with three opponents. Just move around attacking anything within reach without getting sandwiched or blind-sided. After a time your peripheral vision becomes more functional and your hearing as well. Then strategic movement and an enhanced distance sense will begin to come into play. You will find that mobility is truly your friend. You will also discover how critical edge ability helps your mobility and how useful a good sense of the "room" truly is. After a time, most will become quite creative, throwing in kicks and punches, traps and sweeps, etc.

You will not have to create opportunities to work on left-right balancing of your technique. This is inherent in the melee environment. Opponents will be coming at you from all sides and angles. Your experiences on this with a single opponent will soon be honed into a ready, multi-sided combat ability.

You also learn to deal with opponents quickly and decisively. There are always others maneuvering on you, so get the opponent and get away, or just get away, possibly maneuvering the opponent into striking range of someone else as you do so. Thinking quickly in a combat situation is vitally important. This practice helps develop this ability.

If there is room, five or even more opponents can be tried. Our group sometimes has a lurker on the sidelines waiting for an opportunity to try a weapons disarm technique. If successful, he joins the melee and the one who lost the weapon becomes the lurker.

# 6. Additional Practices

As this book evolved, it morphed into a rather different and somewhat longer form than the original basic introduction to the iron ball I had envisioned. Much of this was due to information from the collaborators, my excellent editor, and my training partners. The final order and content of the material presented resulted in a few areas where some elaboration would be good but would require digressing into more detail than was necessary at that point. This section includes material that could not be fitted into the order or subject context. I present it here as a useful and valuable expansion on some important concepts.

## *Practice of Fundamental Technique*

Breaking down the biomechanics of a concept or a technique using the ball as a study aid has been a very rewarding practice.

It is easy to choose a concept of interest, such as the critical edge, reverse abdominal breathing, center application, system integration, etc., and consider it on a very fundamental level along with the biomechanical investigation. If you have problems or questions with some of the concepts, solutions may be found here as well.

Adapting the ball practice to your personal martial arts style would include considerable exploration of fundamental techniques. The possibilities are, of course, endless. Immediately below are a few samples to get you started.

These all assume a critical edge combat posture, but experimentation is the lifeblood of progress, so unbalanced beaten posture or wherever your fancy takes you is certainly fine. Just do not hurt yourself. In all of these fundamental exercises where you are holding the ball, try to feel that the ball is also held in and moved by the pelvic cup.

## Stepping with Reverse Punch

This very basic attacking punch is biomechanically identical to the natural balanced way we walk. This makes it an ideal ball application for studying fundamental technique. The natural cross loading balancing mechanisms cited earlier in the book are already in place, so developing a good feel for effective whole-body movement with good center integration is relatively easy.

Practice the punch with the ball held in both the standing leg and the stepping leg sides from a critical edge combat stance. Start easily with a relatively high stance. Be aware of the internalizing considerations, core energy transfer, center integration, breath management, etc. Your focus is internal, monitoring your biomechanics. A visualized opponent can be added when you feel comfortable with your technique and are raising your intensity level.

Compare the feeling of the technique when the ball is held in the punching side hand with when it is in the withdrawing side hand. Test this with some very moderate resistance, such as a fight shield held lightly by a training partner. Vary the timing of the steps relative to the punch until you feel maximum application of core energy to the target. Work through any other questions regarding the overall concepts with your training partners.

## Kicking with the Ball in the Standing-Leg-Side Hand

This drill is good for studying hip action and middle center usage when executing a front kick. It has the same natural cross-loading balancing biomechanics as the stepping reverse punch and gives insight into integrating the lower center with the middle and upper centers during the kick.

From a combat stance on the critical edge, with the ball held in the front hand, execute a front kick with the back leg while simultaneously reaching out with the ball as though extending your guard a bit. The critical edge stance is established on the opposite side when the kicking leg touches down and the ball simultaneously comes back all the way to the combat hand position, transferring to the other hand on the way. Repeat the kick on the opposite side. Both hand and foot seamlessly retract from final extension without lingering.

Continue the process of alternate side kicking and guarding. Vary the timing of the guard move a bit to note the effect on your biomechanics. If your posture is disturbed, one shoulder raising up, or if your neck muscles are tense, make corrections. The weight of the ball and the middle center action induce the standing leg hip to properly function with the lower center rather than act as part of the upper leg. This common standing leg tendency causes problems for other techniques beside kicks, although it is easily corrected.

Visualize an opponent at slightly differing distances and note that the guard move requires varying timing for optimum results.

Repeat the process without the ball. When it feels okay, work with a partner who maintains a good combat distance while maneuvering evasively and who occasionally tests your guard.

## Stepping with a Front Punch

Like the front kick, the front punch applies stepping-leg-side contact to the opponent and poses the same problem of also applying maximum possible standing leg force into the technique. If this is achieved, a truly effective whole-body, integrated-centers punch follows rather easily. The natural cross loading biomechanical action of the stepping reverse punch is not present, but the same process of withdrawing side, core energy transfer, etc. apply. Practice, especially fight shield training with a partner, will work effectively here.

- - -

The above three techniques can be considered as comprising a practice set that, once familiar, can be used in a fundamental way to work on any nuances of particular interest such as breath management in rebound practice.

## Stepping with a Double Punch

The basic execution of this technique was discussed on page 106. After becoming familiar, it is a good drill to work on with a partner.

Step one is to develop a sudden, fluid explosiveness of the centers through a visualized opponent as described earlier in the book. Basically the technique is executed with the ball held in both hands in a double thrust. The ball should also be held in both the standing leg hand and the stepping leg hand while executing a double hand thrust. Then practice with a visualized ball and finally with truly empty hands.

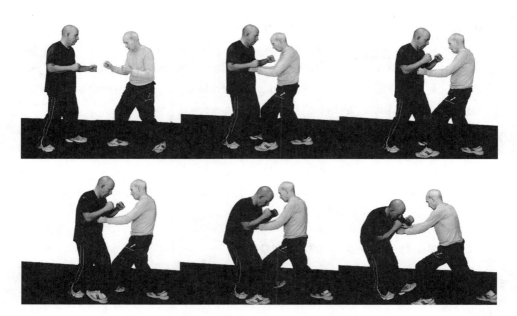

**Figure 84: Stepping with a double punch.**

After some proficiency is acquired, the fundamental technique can be adapted into the basic combat drill shown below.

This drill was developed for a relatively close distance, non-telegraphed, whole-body attack. Both hands go without predetermined roles. On the way, one hand morphs into the attacking role and the other hand into a defensive role or to a supplementary attack according to the changing situation vis-à-vis the opponent. Figure 85, Figure 86, and Figure 87 show many of the possible non-programmed, morphing hand outcomes. A slick opponent may force both hands into defensive roles.

A basic goal is that when and wherever contact with the opponent is made, full force can be transmitted. This is to say that if the opponent closed with you just as you launched, your whole-body movement and dynamic critical edge would enable effective force to be applied to the opponent. This can be effectively studied by training against a fight shield held by a partner who randomly modifies the combat distance with disruptive timing. One way to practice full-force applications is shown in Figure 88.

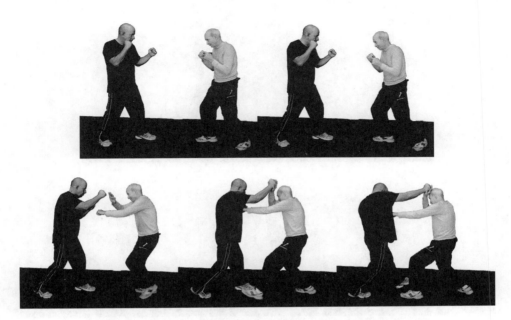

**Figure 85: Non-programmed combat drill, sequence one.**

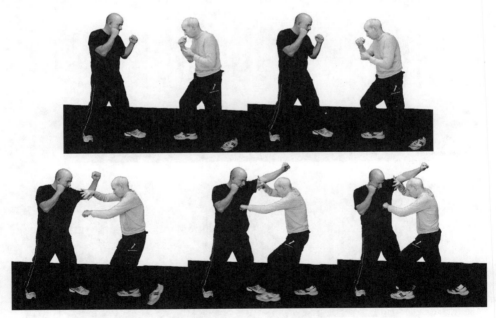

**Figure 86: Non-programmed combat drill, sequence two.**

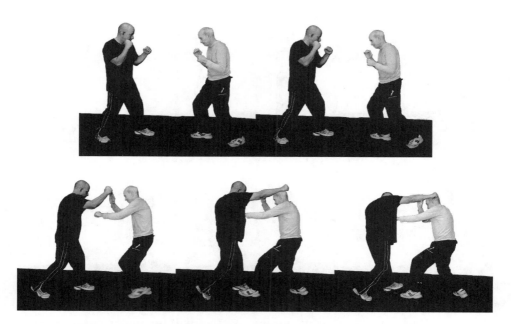

**Figure 87: Non-programmed combat drill, sequence three.**

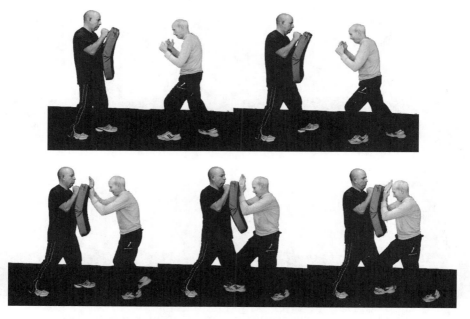

**Figure 88: Practice for applying full force to the opponent.**

## Kicking with Ball and Double Attack

The centers, feet, and hands finish the attack simultaneously inside the visualized opponent. The feeling is that of suddenly stepping onto the opponent while simultaneously reaching into him with both hands. Return to the critical edge is established as the hands instantly return to the combat position and the foot withdraws a bit on the way to touching down.

Practice the basic move, as shown on page 110, with the ball held in both hands and then the standing leg and the stepping (kicking) leg hands. Then add in practice with the visualized ball and the empty hands.

Apparently the idea here is simply to achieve a triple-pronged attack to overwhelm the opponent's defense, probably the eyes, throat, and groin. Actually there are several possibilities with this move. It could also be a smothering defensive move against a suddenly sensed, close range attack. It could be a mixed attacking-defending or attacking-disrupting move.

In any case, the key to success is instant core energy transference onto the opponent, from the critical edge, with good rebound management. This can be practiced and tested in the same manner as the double punch drill above.

# *Breathing*

It is somewhat ironic that something as natural as breathing can, on occasion, be a real distraction when breath integration with unfamiliar technique or concept is required. Breathing is a Big Deal, a critical element of the process of mind-body integration and/or the intent-execution focus of martial artists. My brother Curt remarked once that breathing is one of the few automatic body functions that is easily controlled and managed or, unfortunately, mismanaged. It is important that one properly use one of the various martial arts breathing methods automatically without any distraction from the many other critical concepts and considerations being studied.

All the martial arts abdominal breathing methods work well, so one's starting point will most likely be that of his introductory art. There are, however, several highly desirable nuances of breathing technique that merit serious consideration if they are not already incorporated into your method.

If this incorporation is a distraction from the overall ball study, focusing for a time on breathing exercises appropriate to the personal situation is the obvious solution. Here are some suggestions along that line that worked well for my training partners and me.

## Basic Abdominal Inhalation Breathing

The triple front kick combination described on page 112 is a good introduction for a continuously flowing feeling while working on inhalation/ unregulated breathing.

Next, work on executing techniques, inhaling or exhaling as you execute, using normal abdominal breathing. Move around shadow boxing until you are executing well without disrupting your breathing. Then try light sparring until your breathing is disruption free. The point is to avoid having to program your combat around your breathing.

The ideal time to attack is often described as just when your opponent has finished exhaling. Good luck with that! Controlling distance, timing, breathing, combat line, opponent disinformation, etc. of a truly dangerous opponent is really problematical. Work for the ability to be reasonably effective even if you come out on the short end of the ideal situation. Inhaling in a beaten posture? Still be dangerous.

Try your favorite ball exercises while focusing on the basic abdominal breathing concern. Use various ball weights for this. Use the visualization of the pelvic cup holding the ball as mentioned above. The center of the lower center is the contact point for the ball. As you work and begin to get rather winded, your lower abdominals will really have to extend themselves to move enough air. Breathing becomes much more pronounced, thus greatly enabling your ability to monitor how well you are breathing. Adjustments for even, smooth, unregulated inhalation/exhalation abdominal breathing or for inhalation/exhalation reverse abdominal breathing (immediately below) are then more clearly made.

As with so many concepts, sparring with the flexible weapons and adequate protective equipment is an excellent practical venue for ingraining effective unregulated breathing.

## Reverse Abdominal Breathing

Reverse abdominal breathing was introduced on page 48. Here are some more ideas for practicing it.

Practice walking around while utilizing reverse abdominal breathing when in the normal correct posture. I suggest you use the *Root of Chinese Qigong* book information cited earlier or the Mantak Chia book, if you have it, as your guide in this.

Switch to the combat posture when you are doing okay with the reverse abdominal breathing, then segue into combat maneuvers. Add ball maneuvers (see immediately above) and the forms. Finally, take it out on the track and spar with one of your preferred training partners.

For a truly realistic application, practice of reverse breathing/reverse abdominal breathing during melee sparing, with or without weapons, is ideal.

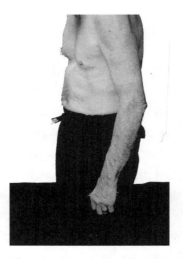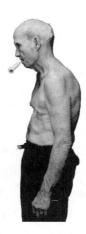

**Figure 89: Reverse abdominal breathing, inhaling with stomach going in, using a resistance-training device.**

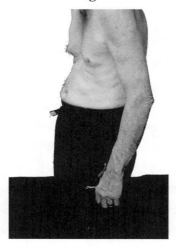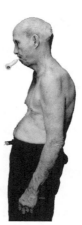

**Figure 90: Reverse abdominal breathing, exhaling with stomach expanding, using a resistance-training device.**

The resistance breath training devices shown in Figure 89 and Figure 90 are available at many diving shops and online from Alimed.com and Amazon.com, among others. They are helpful for jump-starting reverse abdominal breathing technique. This one is called The Breather®.

## *Final Thoughts*

The more familiar you are with the ball, the more rapid your progress will be. Obviously this book is just an introduction to a many-faceted study. Here are a few of the many things you can try. Your martial arts background will surely suggest many other exercises that will be pertinent to your personal goals.

Combining personalization with ball familiarization is a very practical approach. I would suggest that this personalization be considered in terms of the structure, flow, and maneuver presented in this book to maximize its relevancy to the process.

- Be sure to apply the internalizing, breath management, etc. concepts and considerations to the familiarization process.
- If you are right handed, go lefty for a couple of weeks.
- Do your other forms with the iron ball. If you do not do forms, try your common exercises.
- Work with the ball, then hit the bag with and without weapons.
- Just play around with the ball exploring movement, the various concepts, etc. with no fixed final object. Occasionally your creativity will surface and something good will pop into your mind.

- - -

These are some observations that are not within the thrust of the book but are ideas worth thinking about for a martial artist.

- The deeper your anatomical/kinesiological knowledge is, the more accurate your technique insights will be.
- Inefficient or "wrong" techniques (poor biomechanics) executed over time will eventually begin to feel correct and "natural."
- Multiple repetitions of techniques executed with poor biomechanics can really wreck your body.
- You win with your strengths; you lose with your weaknesses.
- No matter how high your level, inevitably, at some point, you will run into a decidedly superior attacker. So, of course, offense is important, but defense, defense, defense.

# Resources

## Books

**Lu Wen Wei, *Illustrated Explanation of Ball Exercises for Health (Nung Wan Jian Shen Tu Shuo)***

Here is an example from the book.

In ancient times the ball was called wan, in modern time's ch'iu. The object itself, however, is one and the same. The first and last forms of this exercise contain/encompass within them a total of thirty-six transformations. All of these transformations, or movements, are based on the semi-circle or arc. Because they make use of the semi-circle they are necessarily followed/shadowed by a formless, non-concrete semi-circle. This then implies the existence of seventy-two transformations. Chuang-Tzu said: its end lacked a tail and its beginning lacked a head. Head and tail being identical, they thus are joined mystically. The large sphere/circle holds within it innumerable and unfathomable small spheres/circles.

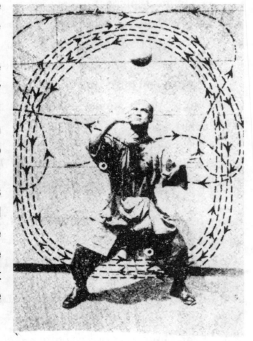

"Seventy-two transformations," "innumerable and unfathomable small spheres/circles" — you can see why I was intrigued but had to simplify things a lot to get started.

**Wan Lai Sheng,** *Compendium of Internal and External Martial Arts (Wushu Nei Wai Gong Zhonghui).*

**Ida Rolf,** *Rolfing, the Integration of Human Structure.* **Harper and Row, 1977.**

**Liang Shou-Yu, Yang Jwing-Ming;** *Hsing Yi Chuan, theory and applications.* **YMAA Publication Center, 1990.**
Hsing Yi is the martial art practiced by Lu Wen Wei's father. This book has excellent information on Wu Chi boxing, three tantiens, chi, yin and yang, and lots more. Really excellent book showing the roots of Lu Wen Wei's thought.

**Gichin Funakoshi,** *Karate-Do Kyohan.* **Kodansha International, 1973.**
For me, the most interesting sections are
- Page 40, three cardinal principles.
- Pages 211, 212 changing hands, transition point.
- Pages 212-223, note the sparring with Mr. Ono operating on the critical edge. Mr. Ono is on the right.
- Maxims for the trainee at the back of the book are well worth reading and pondering.

**Shigeru Egami,** *The Way of Karate* **(1975), republished in a revised edition as** *The Heart of Karate-Do* **by Kodansha America, 2000.**

**Kuo Lien-Ying,** *The T'ai Chi Boxing Chronicle: A Compilation.* **Translated by Guttman, North Atlantic Books, 1994.**
The T'ai Chi boxing terminology is cited in appendix 4.

**Mantak Chia,** *Iron Shirt Chi Kung 1, Healing Tao Books,* **1986.**
A lot of info on chi and qi gong with detailed drills and exercises to develop and control chi. Quite a bit on structure, reverse abdominal breathing, rooting, etc.

Yang Jwing Ming, *The Roots of Chinese Qigong, second edition*. YMAA Publication Center, 1989.

Directions on how to do Daoist reverse abdominal breathing.

Wang Shu Jin, *Bagua book*.

Rick Fields, *The Code of the Warrior*. Harper Collins, 1991.

Martial arts history with information on martial arts mentality and character.

Bruce Lee, *Tao of Jeet Kune Do*. Ohara Publications, 1975.

Although it was not finished, this is a textbook example of analysis, breakdown, and illustration of technique and thought in the martial arts.

Dan Inosanto, *The Filipino Martial Arts*, Know How, 1980.

His first book showing the Philippine combat arts has some excellent historical information and a bunch of other very good stuff. Unfortunately I loaned it out and it did not come back.

Guy Trimble, *Karate Bo, Take-Aways*, Guy Trimble Publishing, 2002.

This rather specialized book shows a staff form, and staff take-aways from several Shotokan style forms. You do not need to be a Shotokan practitioner to appreciate the analysis and realistic understanding of all-out combat presented in the beginning of this book.

Jack Dempsey, *Championship Fighting*, Centerline Press, 1983.

Pages 29-44 are really excellent, showing the falling step and the power line. And there is a lot of other really good stuff throughout the book. If you find this book, do not lend it out.

Thomas Inch, *Spalding's Book on Boxing and Physical Culture*, Gale and Polden Ltd.

This is a very interesting book with a lot of historical boxing, wrestling, and jyu jitsu information.

**Books on Combat Mentality and Training**

**John Cleary, *The Japanese Art of War*, Shambala Publications, 1991.**
This is really excellent on combat mentality training and character development back in the days of the Yagyus, Miyamoto Mushashi, and famous Zen guys. On a side note, the 36 strategies chapter (pages 87-91) is very interesting, like Sun Tzu's *Art of War*. There is another version of them in *The Asian Mind Game* by Chin-Ning Chu.

**The Sword and the Mind, translated with an introduction and notes by Hiroaki Sato. Barnes and Noble Publisher, 2004.**
This book has the Yagyu family traditions in the art of war, the background for it, plus other relevant martial arts information. It has really excellent technical and mentality/character training material on combat and the rationale for it. There is a lot of theoretical and practical combat information including original illustrations. The mentality parts are particularly fine. The historical time line included is valuable and the translator's notes are first-rate (do not overlook them).

**Yagyu Munenori, *The Life-Giving Sword, Secret Teachings from the House of the Shogun,* translated by William Scott Wilson. Kodansha International Ltd., 2003.**
This is the same Yagyu Family Traditions in the Art of War book as the Sato book above with the same content on mental centering, meditation, combat strategy and tactics, illustrations, etc. Being an original English speaker, the translator's comments have a slightly different take on things in some cases. Reading both is worth it.

**Thomas Cleary, *Soul of the Samurai: Modern Translations of Three Classic Works of Zen and Bushido.* Tuttle Publishing, 2005.**
This is the same material as the above two books but with no illustrations. Cleary's commentary is much broader based, making this book well worth studying as well.

**Miyamoto Mushashi,** *The Book of Five Rings*, **translated by Victor Harris. Overlook Press, 1974.**
There is a lot of good discussion of martial arts mentality, strategy, tactics, etc. Miyamoto Mushashi's approach to martial arts was pretty much concerned with winning.

### Books on Biomechanics, Rehabilitation, Etc.

**I. A. Kapandji,** *Physiology of the Joints. Vols. 1, 2 & 3.*
If knowledge of anatomy and physiology is a sideline interest of your martial arts study, these are pictorially exceptional. There is excellent information on the parts of your body that you may be wrecking. They have been around for quite awhile and can be found online for a reasonable price, relatively speaking.

**Eric Franklin,** *Conditioning For Dance*, **Human Kinetics, 2003.**
Good body conditioning and rehab using therabands, soft balls, etc. Very excellent anatomical illustrations help you focus on the precise area in question. Especially good for the pelvic girdle.

## Videos

**Bobby Taboada,** *The Original Art of Balintawak Escrima Cuentada System.* **MATI Productions, Tel 704-392-8410.**
A ten-tape/disk instructional series by this master teacher; principles, concepts, considerations; it's all here.

**Pat Strong,** *Bruce Lee — Lord of Power, Lord of Speed, Lord of Shock, Lord of the Inner Game.*
This four disk/tape set is a comprehensive take on Bruce Lee's Jeet Kune Do from a member of the original Seattle group. It has Bruce Lee's one-inch punch and good information for those whose martial arts did not include a lot of very close range combat.

**Danny Inosanto,** *Tortoise Video.*
This is a very interesting and informative multi-volume overview of the

Philippine martial arts. Lots of drills, tactics, basics, weapons, etc. Vol. 6 has Danny's version of Bruce Lee's one-inch punch.

**Jianye Jiang, *Tai Chi Ball*, Chinese Video Arts Center.**
The tai chi ball material here is very different from the Lu Wen Wei approach but the whole video is quite interesting.

**Dog Brothers. Many videos to choose from.**
These guys do some heavy contact stick fighting and general brawling with minimal protective gear. It is quite intense and exciting to watch.

## Web Sites

There are a ton of websites out there; here are a few of the many that relate to material in this book.

### Wu Ji boxing

Lu Wen Wei trained in Wu Ji boxing and Tai Chi boxing. Wu Ji is less familiar than Tai Chi for most practitioners. Wu Ji is closely associated with Tai Chi and Hsing Yi. It involves standing motionless while completely relaxed and performing some mental exercises.

Under ["wu ji" Chinese boxing] there are a lot of web sites.

"Why is wu ji so important for health?" has an informative write-up under that heading.

"Warriors of stillness" is another such site.

Be sure to put "wu ji" in double quotes or you will get a lot of junk.

### Wan Lai Sheng
**http://www.herner.hu/daniel/shaolin.html**

There are a lot of sites regarding him. I like this one a lot because it has a good deal of other martial information and the Wan Lai Sheng info is substantial, including many pictures, some from my brother's book.

**http://www.sifuchenying.com/wanlaishen.stml**

Information on Wan Lai Sheng and the Zi Ran Men style.

**Ancient Chuo Jiao**

YouTube has four segments of extremely interesting Ancient Chuo Jiao material showing the art of the "penetrating kick." This seems to be really genuine, insightful, old-time martial arts practice. Under YouTube martial arts put "Ancient Chuo Jiao" in quotes/

**Bobby Taboada**

Worldbalintawak.com

    Balintawak Arnis Escrima information.

**Gary Lam Wing Chun**

http://www.garylamwingchun.com/

    Information about Wing Chun as practiced by Gary Lam.

**Lamon Brewster**

www.lamonbrewster.com

**Shot put Sources**

    There are over a hundred sources cited at google.com under track and field shot put sources. Samples of these are

    Wolverine sports: www.school-tech.com/track28.html

    Dowdle sports: dowdlesports.com

    Joe's Sports, Outdoors, and More: www.joessports.com

# Appendices

1. Lu Wen Wei Ball Book translation
2. Wan Lai Sheng ball training exercises
3. The 72 essential terms of the Chinese boxing art
4. Iron ball training testimonials

## Appendix 1. Ball Book Translation

Excerpts from Lu Wen Wei's *Illustrated Explanation of Ball Exercises for Health (Nung Wan Jian Shen Tu Shuo)*.

My father was very disciplined regarding physical culture and never tired of constant training. He had a large number of wooden and metal balls on a rack, The large ones about a foot in diameter, the middle ones five or six inches and the small ones three to four inches. I also trained with them for three to four years, morning and night and never tired of them. As a young man my father trained Xing Yi boxing and from this training derived two techniques which he applied to ball training, zan and fan.

What are zan and fan? Zan is active; fan is quiescent. What are yin and yang? Zan is yang; fan is yin. Zan starts from the inward and then goes outward and up. Fan comes from the outward and then goes inward and down. In all moves the hands and face are toward each other. When the palm is toward the face this is yang; when the back of the hand is toward the face this is yin. The body has three dantian, upper, middle and lower. The arm has three joints, wrist, elbow and shoulder. The hands move in all possible manners scribing large circles of 360 degrees; small circles also have 360 degrees. The large circles are slow, the small circles are fast. Some are shaped; others are formless. In all movements the arms are not straightened and most commonly are bent 90 degrees. This makes the circles lively.

Some years ago I commenced training in Wu Ji boxing and Tai Ji boxing and as my training progressed I began to use the ball to replace the hand techniques. I devised twelve patterns that initiate with zan and then become fan and another 24 patterns that initiate with fan and change to zan. In this book the first twelve patterns are zan; the final 24 are fan.

3.1 As for the hand methods, first there is zan; next there is fan; the third is the arc — they are all mutually dependant. Zan is one hand palm up and pressing upward. The other hand is palm down and pressing downward. All things are subsumed under yin and yang. As soon as Tai Ji moves, yin and yang are distinguished. In the human body the navel is the center. The feet are below, the hands above.

3.5 The navel constitutes the tracks wherein Tai Ji passes through. Consequently if skills are not applied there is no separation of Yin and Yang. The hands and feet are divided into upper and lower and each has both yin and yang movements. As for zan, the one hand is palm up while the other is always palm down. When it changes so that the fingers of one hand are opposite the wrist of the other hand it is still yang.

4.1 Going slightly past when the two hands are back to back, then it becomes yin.

4.2 As for fan, it is when the zan method hand reverses.

## Appendix 2. Wan Lai Sheng Mu Zi Ball Exercises

Mu (literally mother) and zi (literally child) ball: These are primarily conditioning and strengthening exercises and to help develop penetrating power using 18- and 22-pound balls. Do not use hard force.

Grabbing: using only the fingers, practice grabbing the ball. Do not lift the ball completely and do not make contact with the center of the palm.

Lift and twist: grab the ball palm down and, as you lift it, twist the forearm outward. Repeat, alternating the hands.

Flicking the ball: practice slapping and flicking the ball with your fingers.

Pointing: practice tapping the ball with your fingertips (your fingers should be slightly bent to protect your joints and meridians).

Pushing the ball and drilling: practice stabbing the ball with your fingertips. You make contact slightly off center and allow the fingers to slide off to the side. The feeling should be like stabbing forward to attack and drilling through. This practice is to increase your penetrating power.

Knocking: knock or tap the ball with your knuckles, paying particular attention to the knuckles of the first two fingers. You can also condition the smaller knuckles of the whole hand.

Chopping: use the knife-edge of the hand to chop the ball.

Chopping and sliding: again chop the ball, but this time your hand contacts off center and practices sliding through in order to develop penetrating power in a sideways direction.

Lifting and catching: lift the ball with one hand, throw it in the air and catch it with the other hand; repeat alternating the hands.

## Appendix 3. The 72 essential terms of the Chinese boxing art.

The following list of terms was compiled by Kuo Lien Ying, a well-known master of the Guang Ping style of Tai Chi Chuan. It is found in his book, *The T'ai Chi Boxing Chronicle*, translated by Guttman. This list is part of a comprehensive treatment of the Guang Ping style and many of the terms are applicable to other styles of Tai Chi Chuan as well. For information on Kuo Lien Ping and the Guang Ping style there are various books and internet sites available.

These terms are indicative of the many complexities facing an internal martial arts practitioner. The terms cover the various energies, principles, concepts, and potential flaws that make up the core training of Guang Ping Tai Chi Boxing. They are included here not as a teaching tool but as objects for the inquisitive martial artist to examine in searching out ways to enhance his or her own training.

Generally, a specialty of any kind has a vocabulary that illustrates how the system is used. The language of this art is paramount to a complete understanding of the subject matter. A word is a symbol of an idea. If the word and the meaning are not specific and clear, it is difficult to understand this art. You must pass through many years of being taught and studying. Then the terms will become certain and fixed. When you learn the language of Tai Chi boxing, and the meaning of the terms is not clear, then it is not easy to receive the proper vitality from the fixed movements. In order to pass down the mystery of the specific terms, algebra should be used instead of arithmetic. It takes years to get. One can say this is old-fashioned because you cannot escape the fact that the more errors, the more distant the goal. Don't deviate from the boxing art's main theme. Today there is much doubt about the meaning of Tai Chi boxing's terminology. If the basic terms are not understood, eventually it will be like groping for the meaning in a mist. One needs to be exact and specific in order to proceed.

Then an error in the center will not be an error of a thousand miles at the circumference. The terms are explained as follows:

1.  Peng ching — The energy of flexibility and resilience. It is the practice of Ch'i Kung strung together inside. It makes the body like a spring or rubber band.
2.  Lu ching — The energy of friction and rubbing. It is shifting the direction of Peng ching inside and down, causing the direction of Peng and Lu to be mutually attached or corresponding.
3.  Chi ching — This is the energy of two forces combined and changes the direction of Peng. Both hands usually work together and it is a releasing out energy.
4.  An ching — Pressing down with the hands and not disconnecting. It is being fixed to a point on the opponent. It is used to cause a reaction by the opponent and does not cause him to fall directly.
5.  Tsai ching — The energy of two forces divided. It is grasping a point on the opponent so that he cannot issue forth a strike. It is a method of connecting and stopping the opponent from slipping away.
6.  Lieh ching — This is striking energy. During revolving it is collecting great flexibility and then striking out. It is entering the opponent.
7.  Chou ching — This is the elbow striking by moving the arms up and down. It is using Lieh's second line of defense.
8.  Kao ching — A strike by the whole body to upset the energy of the opponent's body. It is using Lieh's third line of defense.
9.  Adhere energy — This is being fixed to one point on the opponent and not moving from it. It is like taking root on this point. Regardless of what changes occur, you adhere to this point.
10. Stick energy — To be like glue when moving. It is to be fixed to one part of the opponent close and tight. Whatever the movement, you do not move from this surface.

11. Connecting energy — In retreating you have pulling energy. You extend the opponent's energy towards the inside of your circle and grab.
12. Following energy — In entering it has the energy of pushing. It is your energy extending into the opponent's circle and striking.
13. Empty energy — Draining an opponent's energy. When he inclines towards you, it drains his energy and makes him stumble.
14. Bind energy — It is supporting or aiding another's energy. It is using the opponent's stiff energy and supporting it with your own energy. Your energy supports in two directions while tightly attached to his body and allows you to pull.
15. Break energy — Energy which turns towards the inside and down. Its posture wraps inside. It is empty draining energy and prevents the opponent from getting a good position.
16. Rubbing energy — Energy which turns away outside and up. Its posture is outside and away. It is a dissipating energy and prevents the opponent from getting a good position.
17. Tangle energy — A screwing action which circles around the opponent. It revolves around a fixed point and does not let the opponent get away.
18. Receiving energy — Extending your own energy and giving it length. You evenly receive another's energy and continue to lengthen.
19. Stirring energy — Like the joining of the bamboo shoot, the energy is inside. It is continuously receiving the opponent's energy and completely forming this corresponding line.
20. Rousing energy — This is sudden and shocking. The whole body rolls, collects, and afterwards suddenly strikes.
21. Twisting energy — The body turns sideways. It is the turning of the body that changes the energy. It is not hard or stiff and does not resist.

22. Returning energy — The inside spirals or twists and the outside does the returning. It is a grasping energy which does not stop during return or release.

23. Provoking energy — Induces an energy to emerge. It is a revolving pressure which causes a reaction.

24. Grabbing energy — A snatching of the joints using the fingers. The opponent's body is partially caged through bone locking.

25. Exchange energy — This is shifting with partial energy and exchanging the energy of the joints. You greatly open the opponent's joints and change him.

26. Concluding energy — Suddenly releasing and showing energy. This is to catch someone off guard when there is a gap between bodies. Then enter and strike without separating. Lieh, Releasing, and Striking.

27. Taking energy — Another gives you his energy. It is the opponent's energy which comes. The rolling and releasing is calm and smooth.

28. Giving energy — The opponent receives your energy. Never be stingy but send it out firmly, sink down, and give.

29. Rolling energy — The large circle changes to the small circle. One uses the spiral from the large to the small circle.

30. Releasing energy — The small circle changes to the large circle. One uses the outward spiral from the small to the large circle.

31. Collecting energy — This is the energy of the bow. It is adding in Peng ching and rolling and releasing so that the bow is ready to fire.

32. Striking energy — Its nature is sudden and straight. It comes from the release of flexibility and strikes out. It can be Lieh or Releasing.

33. The two concepts — They are of equal importance when meeting strength. They are outward and inward drawing of

silk's reciprocal use. This is the achievement of meeting strength.

34. Empty-Solid — A deviation of the center of gravity. The center of gravity is stable while the body is active. This deviation of the center of gravity is what allows activity.

35. The scale — The body stands upright without leaning in any direction.

36. Stationary point — With the vertical comes the horizontal station. With the horizontal comes the vertical station.

37. Defect — The Ch'i is not full. Some part of the body is lacking in Peng ching.

38. Yin-Yang — The two are different yet work together. It is releasing, out, striking, opening, hard, meat, use, Ch'i, body, action, and receiving, in, collecting, closing, soft, bone, foundation, reason, mind, and stillness.

39. Listening energy — Waiting for the opponent to express energy. Wait for his slightest movement and move first by following.

40. Opportunity — If there is opportunity you can succeed. It is getting the opportunity to enter the opponent.

41. The Position — The center of gravity is stable. It is not overextending the two feet yet deviating the center of gravity. Then you are smooth and active.

42. Open-Extend — Adding a large movement to the circle. It is expanding the body from the interior.

43. Close-Contract — Adding a small movement to the circle. It is the degree of contracting the body. It is the Ch'i moving the body.

44. Eight trigrams — They are the eight energy separations. It is during movement that the energies have different positions.

45. Five elements — They are the direction of the five steps.

46. Folding — If something is up it must come from below. If you want to move something up it starts from below.

47. Borrowing strength — Adding speed by following an opponent's direction and adding speed by pulling or following.
48. Ch'i Kung — The oxygen in the blood is regulated by adding Ch'i. It is directed by the will power and moves in an orbit.
49. Pulling — Sinking and changing to dragging or pulling. You utilize the energy of sinking down, which measures the strike. Everything is drawn toward the outside.
50. Outward drawing of silk — Revolves toward the outside and up. It is attacking drawing of silk used to force another's energy.
51. Inward drawing of silk — Revolves toward the inside and down. It is defensive drawing of silk and is used to drain another's energy.
52. Bones receive the bamboo shoot — This is getting the point of centrifugal force and then striking the opponent's center of gravity.
53. Movement changes who is in charge — Using centrifugal force, all movements from the waist and spine are focused on a central point. It changes the other's energy.
54. Spirit/Ch'i boil — The spirit and Ch'i are lively and aroused. This occurs during moving energy. The Ch'i follows the spirit, the spirit follows the intention, and all movements are enhanced.
55. Upper and lower united — The hands and feet are divided into empty and solid. It is the relationship of the hands and feet; when the left hand is empty the right foot is solid, and when the left hand is solid the right foot is empty.
56. The whole body is one unit — The entire body is strung together and continuously moves together. When the body moves, no part remains still.
57. Collecting into the bones — The spirit and Ch'i are concealed inside. It is the idea of the tendons lengthening and moving.

58. Awareness energy — Knowing yourself and knowing the enemy. This is to know the opponent's energy and changes and all of his actions.

59. The two shoulders are joined — The two arms are connected by a line between the shoulders. Move one back, the other moves forward.

60. The legs follow each other — The two legs are connected. This gives them flexibility. When one leg moves, the other must follow.

61. Empty dexterity's top energy — The top of the head has Peng ching. The top is suspended and connected by a line from the top of the head to the middle of the waist.

62. Sinking shoulders, drooping elbows — Don't let the shoulders and elbows rise. Make the elbows sink downward and then the shoulders will sink down also.

63. Contain the chest, pull up the back — Don't make the chest convex or concave. Don't make the chest large. It is the idea of the spine drawn up straight, then the front of the chest is contained.

64. Loosen the waist, open the hips — The waist is like a belt which revolves. It revolves when the body is upright, then the waist can relax.

65. Top defect — The top is overextended in some direction. Then the Peng ching is lacking and you can be bumped or pushed.

66. Stiffness defect — The degree of Peng ching is insufficient. There is no liveliness in more than one direction.

67. Trying to get rid of the opponent defect — This is letting go of the point on the opponent. Losing contact with the opponent will hinder flexibility. The opponent should be close, not far away.

68. The defect of resisting — The response is too distant and too early. Follow the opponent, don't resist.

69. Leaning forward defect — If the front of the body leans forward, this harms the waist energy. It causes the center of gravity to fall forward.

70. Leaning backward defect — When the body leans backward, it causes the chest to protrude. Again, the center of gravity is upset.

71. Breaking off defect — This is breaking off and not remaining in contact with the opponent. It is similar to resisting.

72. Receiving defect — One appears to be receiving but is not. If one receives straight, directly and solidly, it is not using the idea of the wheel.

The above seventy-two definitions are Tai Chi boxing's most frequently used terms. The definitions are useful for understanding the Tai Chi boxing system. One must study and contemplate deeply in order to be sure that the correct meaning matches the definition. This will prevent the student from straying from the main road. Progress in this skill is slow, and you must labor ardently to understand the objective of this boxing method. The results one gets from practice are seriously connected with the understanding of the above definitions. Study the source of these terms with diligence and translate their meanings because these are boxing's essentials. The purpose of these terms is to contain them within your body, but without these terms as a standard criterion, the basic points will only be general and not completely clear. Without the terms, your activity appears to be but is not Tai Chi boxing.

# Appendix 4. Iron ball training testimonials

**Lamon Brewster (WBO heavyweight boxing champion, April 2004 to April 2006):**

I was introduced to the iron ball training techniques by Tom Muzila. In my training I always put a huge amount of focus on the amount of power I could acquire from my punches. I was able to develop a decent amount of power in my punches through the years. I couldn't believe the extra amount of penetration power I was able to attain with my punches after Tom trained and introduced me to the iron ball techniques.

**Tom Muzila:**

I trained and introduced Lamon Brewster to these unique iron ball training techniques early in his professional career. I learned and was taught them by my first karate instructor, Caylor Adkins, years ago. Lamon already had a significant amount of power in his punches. After training Lamon a short time with the iron ball, his body quickly started moving more efficiently. His hips, punches, and body moved more as one unit. His punching power increased to be more remarkable than it already was. I would wholeheartedly recommend these iron ball training techniques to any martial artist, karate practitioner, or boxer.

# Index

# About the Author

Caylor Adkins, now 76 years old, began his martial arts practice in October 1957 at John Ogden's judo and karate school in Compton, California. He has practiced continuously with dedication since that time.

He was an early student of Tsutomu Ohshima, founder of Shotokan Karate of America (SKA). As part of the SKA, he was a member of the team that assisted Mr. Ohshima in the translation of Shotokan Master Gichin Funakoshi's book (*Karate-Do Kyohan*) into English. Mr. Adkins served as SKA president for many years and is currently a member of the SKA senior advisory council. He attained the highest rank that is awarded in SKA, that of fifth degree black belt, in 1976.

He was a frequent contributor to *Black Belt* and *Karate Illustrated* magazines in the 1960s and 1970s. His contributions included technical articles and also articles regarding sport karate and its involvement with the Amateur Athletic Union (AAU) and the World Union of Karate-do Organizations (WUKO). In those organizations he served as National Chairman of the AAU karate committee (1975-1977) and as first vice president of WUKO (1975-1977). He also chaired the organizing committee for the 1975 World Karate-do Championship Tournament held in Long Beach, California.

Known as a devotee of rigorous training with a bias for combat he has always sought broadly based sources of instruction for himself including the influences from the following martial arts practitioners:

Tsutomu Ohshima, Shotokan Karate
John Ogden, judo
Shigeru Egami, Shotokai Karate
Harold Gunns, western boxing
Dave and Chris Shaver, western boxing
Pat Strong, Jeet Kune Do
Bobby Taboada, Balintawak Cuentada Escrima
Hironori Ohtsuka, Wadokai Karate
Huang Wen Shan, Yang style Tai Chi Chuan

He is currently retired and living in Pittsburgh, Pennsylvania, with his wife Carol and two cats, Thelma and Louise. His practice continues with breaks for exploring Pittsburgh and reading science fiction and mystery novels.